ANTI INFLAMMATORY DIET FOR BEGINNERS

HEAL YOUR BODY FROM WITHIN TROUGHT THIS ULTIMATE PROVEN GUIDE TO ACTIVATE AUTOPHAGY FOR ANTI-AGING AND WEIGHT LOSS

[Ashla Mittal]

Text Copyright © [Ashla Mittal] 2020

All rights reserved. No part of this guide may be reproduced in any form without permission in writing from the publisher except in the case of brief quotations embodied in critical articles or reviews.

Legal & Disclaimer

The information contained in this book and its contents is not designed to replace or take the place of any form of medical or professional advice; and is not meant to replace the need for independent medical, financial, legal or other professional advice or services, as may be required. The content and information in this book has been provided for educational and entertainment purposes only.

The content and information contained in this book has been compiled from sources deemed reliable, and it is accurate to the best of the Author's knowledge, information and belief. However, the Author cannot guarantee its accuracy and validity and cannot be held liable for any errors and/or omissions. Further, changes are periodically made to this book as and when needed. Where appropriate and/or necessary, you must consult a professional (including but not limited to your doctor, attorney, financial advisor or such other professional advisor) before using any of the suggested remedies, techniques, or information in this book.

Upon using the contents and information contained in this book, you agree to hold harmless the Author from and against any damages, costs, and expenses, including any legal fees potentially resulting from the application of any of the information provided by this book. This disclaimer applies to any loss, damages or injury caused by the use and application, whether directly or indirectly, of any advice or information presented, whether for breach of contract, tort, negligence, personal injury, criminal intent, or under any other cause of action.

You agree to accept all risks of using the information presented inside this book.

You agree that by continuing to read this book, where appropriate and/or necessary, you shall consult a professional (including but not limited to your doctor, attorney, or financial advisor or such other advisor as needed) before using any of the suggested remedies, techniques, or information in this book.

Table of Contents

Introduction — 6

CHAPTER 1: AUTOPHAGY, WHAT IS IT? — 8
    The Process of Autophagy — 12
    The Function of Autophagy — 14
    Xenophagy — 14
    Nutrient Starvation — 14
    Infection — 15
    Programmed Cellular Death — 15
    Repair Mechanism — 16

CHAPTER 2: THE SECRETS OF AUTOPHAGY — 17
    Autophagy Mechanisms — 20
    When Autophagy Goes Wrong — 22
    Understand the Difference Between Psychological and Physical Hunger — 25
    My Experience — 26
    Take Tea or Coffee Without Adding Sugar — 28
    Ensure You're Drinking Plenty of Water — 29
    Go to Bed — 30
    Distract Yourself — 32
    Flee from Places Where You Can Smell or See Food — 35
    Meditate — 37
    Remember Why You Started — 37
    Habit Changes — 38

CHAPTER 3: THE BENEFITS OF AUTOPHAGY — 39
    Side Effects of Fasting — 44
    Precautions to Take When Fasting — 46

CHAPTER 4: HOW AUTOPHAGY MAY IMPROVE THE QUALITY AND LENGTH OF YOUR LIFE — 48
    Start Fasting Gradually — 51

Eating the Right Foods	52
Exercise Suggestions For You	57
The Significance of Sleep While Fasting	60
Professional GuidanceDuring Water-Fasting	60
How A Chiropractor Will Help With The Fasting Process	62

CHAPTER 5: REGULATION OF INFLAMMATION AND IMPROVED MUSCLE PERFORMANCE BY AUTOPHAGY   64

Risks and Cautions of Performance Autophagy	69

CHAPTER 6: AUTOPHAGY IMPROVES YOUR SKIN HEALTH AND MINIMIZES APOPTOSIS (CELL -DEATH)   74

How to Induce Autophagy	76
Autophagy Fasting	79
Water-Fasting, Autophagy, and Anti-Aging The Intersection	82

CHAPTER 7: WHAT ACTIVATES AUTOPHAGY?   83

Ways to Initiate Autophagy	87
Intermittent Water Fasting	89
Exercise	90
Ketosis	100
Insulin and Ketosis	101
Fasting	106
Intermittent Water Fasting	111

CHAPTER 8: HEAL YOUR BODY FROM WITHIN   114

How To Make Fasting A Way of Life?	114

CHAPTER 9: WEIGHT LOSS   124

CHAPTER 10: FEELING GOOD   127

CONCLUSION   130

Introduction

Unfortunately, the food of today is focused more on caloric value than nutritional value, and the worst part is that we are too exposed to it. Finding organic food in urban areas is quite a difficult task, as pesticides are used on fruits, chemical fertilizers are used on vegetables and other legumes, and animals are being fed concentrated food before being slaughtered. This is how a chicken grows so fast, but this affects also other animals. All of these factors influence the quality of our food and may lead to several diseases, especially related to high blood sugar levels. Diabetes was not a very common disease a few centuries ago, but now it's amongst the most spread diseases worldwide. Heart, kidney or liver diseases are very common, but also neurodegenerative diseases like Alzheimer's or Parkinson's disease are becoming more and more "popular." How we can reverse all of these and put a stop to it? Is medication a solution? Medication is not designed to cure, but instead, it was designed to make the disease a bit more pleasant by masking the symptoms. In a positive scenario, it can only stimulate the body to overcome the disease. The body heals itself, so why use a medicine, especially when it comes to common conditions and diseases like high blood sugar and insulin, heart, kidney and liver diseases.

Autophagy is the answer to all these problems, and in this book, you can learn how you can activate it and what benefits it has. In this book, you will discover different methods on how to induce or activate autophagy. Although some of them may sound discouraging, you can find in here important tips on how to practice these methods, how to maximize their effects and of course, the benefits of each method. You can discover important information about Intermittent Fasting, Ketosis, HIIT and Protein Fast. The cure for all of the diseases mentioned above is within your grasp, and the best part is that you don't have to pay serious cash for medicine. After reading this book, you will think again before buying medicine for such diseases and therefore save a lot of money. Autophagy is not holistic or "voodoo" medicine, it is something real, something that won the Nobel prize a few years ago, so it's a practice that you should take it very seriously. There are plenty of reasons why you should consider getting your body into autophagy mode, and you can find all of them if you read the chapters of this book.

CHAPTER 1: AUTOPHAGY, WHAT IS IT?

The word "autophagy" is derived from the Ancient Greek word, meaning "hollow" or "self-devouring." It may sound ominous, but it is a natural process in your body to help you regulate the various cellular components you need and do not need for proper functioning. It is descriptive of the process of regulation, and how your body breaks down cells if they are dysfunctional or unnecessary. Those parts that are removed are then recycled or properly disposed of so you can have a healthy body. It is an orderly process or degradation and dissolution.

There are three primary types of autophagy, which occur in your body: chaperone-mediated autophagy, or CMA; microautophagy, and; macroautophagy. Each type has a unique role and purpose in your body. When you are sick or have a disease, your body's response to this stress, which is your body's natural survival instinct, is a response that adapts to the problem at hand. Because of its adaptability, it will either show up and help kill or destroy cells or break them apart to try to restore them. At times, the process can appear to support the morbidity of the affected cells. In cases where your body becomes extremely starved, the natural autophagy process will breakdown parts of cells to help the cell survive on less energy, leading to the best chance of survival. They remove the "unnecessary" components at the moment to help the cells keep up their energy levels.

In 1963, when Dr. Christian de Duve discovered the function of the body's lysosomes, he coined the name, "autophagy." Later, in the 1990s, researchers studying yeast found autophagic-like properties, which lead to the discovery of the process. A Nobel Peace Prize in Physiology or Medicine was awarded in 2016 to Yoshinori Ohsumi, a Japanese researcher who was prominent in the 1990s autophagy deduction. Prior to all of this, in 1962, Keith Porter and a student first observed the process of autophagy at Rockefeller Institute. They identified the lysosome quantity was increased in rat's livers after glucagon was introduced. They observed how some moved to the center of the cells but had a severe flaw in their interpretation—they did not consider the organelles that already existed and the formation of the lysosome. Their name, "autolysis" was coined after Christian de Duve and Alex Novikoff's work, but it was not accurate. This is why de Duve was credited with the discovery in 1963. Christian de Duve began his work after being introduced to a study published in early 1963 by Hruban, Spargo and their colleagues. Their publication described "focal cytoplasm degradation." This observation and study were based off a German study from 1955 studying injuries. Their observations launched de Duve's own inquiry, which ultimately leads to his coining of the process as "autophagy." Not making the same conclusion as Porter and his student, de Duve observed that the function of the lysosome was influenced by the glucagon, but it was a major part of the cellular degradation in the liver of the subjects. During this study, de Duve and his student Russell Deter explained that lysosomes were the reasons for the autophagy caused by glucagon. This is the first moment that lysosomes were described as the center for intracellular autophagy.

After Ohsumi received his award for his work with autophagy, the field grew dynamically throughout the 21st century. Several studies were conducted on the subject, shedding light on new tools for scientists to learn about human's response to disease and their general health. In 1999, Beth Levine and her group of researchers made an incredible discovery that altered the course of autophagy and researchers ever since. Levine and her group identified a strong connection between autophagy and cancer. Even today, the main research topic of autophagy relates to cancer. Another common theme in research is the relationship between immune defense and neurodegeneration. In 2003, the first Gordon Research Conference in Waterville focused on autophagy. Later, in 2005, Daniel Klionsky published a scientific journal focused on autophagy, titled "Autophagy." In 2007, the first Keystone Symposia and Conference held in Monterey was dedicated to autophagy. Research continues to unfold new and interesting applications of understanding about autophagy and its role in the human body.

The Process of Autophagy

All three types of autophagy are facilitated by genes related to autophagy and related enzymes. Because of the size of macroautophagy, it is further divided into "selective" and "bulk" macroautophagy. "Selective" refers to organelle autophagy. This includes ribophagy, coprophagy, pexophagy, lipophagy, and mitophagy. The main type of autophagy in a person's body is Macroautophagy. The primary purpose is to remove damaged organelles from cells or proteins that are not in use. The process works like this: the phagophore selects the items that need to be removed and it surrounds them. This creates an autophagosome, or a double membrane, surrounding the selected organelle or protein. The autophagosome then makes its way through the cell's cytoplasm until it reaches a lysosome. When it finds one, and the two bind together. The autophagosome enters into the lysosome and begins to degrade because of the lysosomal hydrolase.

Other times, the autophagy is more direct, which is known as Microautophagy. The cytoplasm material is engulfed directly into the lysosome. The lysosomal membrane folds inward or is a cellular protrusion called "invagination." A more complex process than the other two is the CMA, or "chaperone-mediated autophagy." The pathway is very specific and involves recognition by an hsc70-containing complex. Basically, this means that when hsc70 complex is present, a protein must have a site that will recognize it. This recognition allows the complex to bind to it, creating CMA-substrate/chaperone complex. This complex then is able to bind to a protein bound for the membrane of the lysosome through the CMA receptor of the protein. This allows the complex to enter the cell. Once inside, the protein unfolds and is sent through the membrane with the help of the hsc70 chaperone. This process is significantly different, mainly because of the translocation of the protein material in a singular manner. It is also an extremely selective process, only allowing very specific material to cross over the barrier of the lysosome.

Two processes related to Macroautophagy include lipophagy and mitophagy. Lipophagy occurs in both fungus and animals. Autophagy can degrade lipids. In plants, this process is not identifiable yet. Lipid Droplets, or LDs, are the targets. These little spheres are the center of most triacylglycerols, or TAGs, and are also a single layer of protein for a membrane and phospholipids. This process was observed and defined in 2009 during a study on mice. The other process, mitophagy, is a result of autophagy. When autophagy does its "job," mitochondria can experience selective degradation. This is most commonly observed when the mitochondria are stressed or damaged, making it defective. This process encourages mitochondrial turnover and also stops the dysfunctional mitochondria from piling up. If too much-damaged mitochondria accumulate the cell can begin to degrade. Even if there are healthy mitochondria present alongside dysfunctional mitochondria, the process is still applied to all present in the cell.

The Function of Autophagy

There are several functions of autophagy, including Xenophanes, nutrient starvation, infection, programmed cell death, and repair mechanisms. Autophagy is present in a variety of cellular functions for a variety of reasons. Below is a brief synopsis of these functions and how autophagy is involved.

Xenophagy

When an infectious particle enters the body, there is degradation caused by autophagy. This is a term most often applied and found in microbiology. In addition to breaking down an infected particle, this almost-mechanical process of autophagy in your cells is critical to helping your immune system. For example, if your body is attached by an intracellular pathogen such as the bacterium that causes tuberculosis, Mycobacterium tuberculosis, the mechanics and mechanisms that choose what mitochondria to degrade are also responsible for degrading this pathogen.

Nutrient Starvation

Autophagy is present at high levels in yeasts when there is nutrient starvation. This is necessary because the unnecessary proteins are degraded and recycled amino acids are used to synthesize the protein to keep your body alive. An example of this process being present is when an animal severs its ties with its trans-placental food supply after birth. Often in a body that is rich in nutrients form mutant cells of yeast that stop the autophagy process, but when those nutrients deplete, so do these mutant cells. When a body enters into starvation, this process is necessary to help keep the body alive as long as possible. It has been shown in studies with mice and is essential for vacuoles protein degradation when starving.

Infection

Your body has intracellular "danger" receptors, such as Galectin-8, which roam your body looking for trouble. When these receptors sense something is attacking the body, like vesicular stomatitis virus, they begin autophagy on the intracellular pathogens. Galectin-8, for example, binds to the critical vacuole and calls for an autophagy adaptor, like NDP52. This then begins the development of an autophagosome and the degradation of the bacteria.

Programmed Cellular Death

PCD, or "programmed cellular death," is related to the look of the autophagosome and relies on the protein in autophagy. This often is associated with a specific process, which is now called "autophagic PCD." There is still debate, much like the "chicken and the egg," about whether cell death caused this process or if this process caused the death of the cell. The process could be an attempt to repair the cell, or an attempt to stop cellular death, or it could be the reason the cell is dying. To this day, there are no histochemical or morphological studies that show the cause in the relationship between the death of the cell and the activity of autophagy in it. What was previously the favored opinion, that autophagy was actually causing the cells to die, has fallen in popularity as more evidence leans towards the possibility of the process trying to save the cell. For example, some arguments present insect metamorphosis as an example of a form of PCD that shows how the cells can be saved instead of killed. It is a distinct cellular change that no other example has shown. After a viral infection, the degree, and type of stress that signals for regulation can determine the chances of a cell of survival or death. These recent studies still need more research to show this relationship; however, the biochemical and pharmacological results are promising.

Repair Mechanism

The reason you age is that your body stops removing damaged cells, but rather allows them to accumulate in your body. This is why you begin to get wrinkles and your muscles begin to breakdown. Degeneration of autophagy is credited as one of the reasons for this cellular accumulation. This is because a working autophagic process breaks down the dysfunctional proteins, cell membranes, and organelles. If your body decides to no longer use this process, you begin to start aging. When there are lysosomal damage autophagy receptors, like by "directors" Galectin-8 and Galectin-3, and autophagy is present. When this is triggered, galectins often call for help from other receptors like NDP52 and TRIM16. This also directly impacts AMPK and mTOR activity in your body. AMPK and mTOR, on the other hand, activate and also inhibit autophagy respectively in your body.

CHAPTER 2: THE SECRETS OF AUTOPHAGY

Phagaphore is the "hallmark" of the autophagy process. It is a double-membrane structure that moves around. Unlike secretory transport vesicles that separate from an organelle carrying "cargo" inside already, the phagophore picks up its load while it is assembling. The sequential expansion allows the phagophore to take on a little load or a large load. There is a lot of flexibility in how much they can carry. When it expands to load in something, it separates the cytoplasmic parts, including other, complete organelles, lipids, and proteins. As soon as it is loaded, it closes and turns into an autophagosome. Once matured into the autophagosome, the cargo remains contained in the lumen. Through-membrane fusion the autophagosome delivers its load to the lytic compartments. In plants and fungi, this is vacuole and in metazoans it is lysosomes. Once there, the cargo is degraded and recycled.

It is possible to see autophagy broadly categorized into two categories—nonselective and selective. It is categorized by what is being picked up or "eaten." When studied more extensively, it is broken down further into macroautophagy, microautophagy, and CMA, or chaperone-mediated Autophagy, as described in the previous chapter. In order for the cells in your body to be in balance or in homeostasis, autophagy must be present and functioning properly. In addition, autophagy is necessary for cellular survival when your body is stressed, such as when it is nutrient deficient. The process of autophagy is upregulated. This means that the degradation and sequestering of parts of the cell are determined by the severity of the situation. Once it arrives and assesses the "damage," the process returns macromolecules into the cytosol. This is essential to the metabolic reaction of the cell and generates power and energy.

The process of autophagy is precisely orchestrated and tightly regulated. The pathological and physiological role it plays in your body is essential, as evidenced by its support in the health of your cells both when your body is under stress, like starvation or infection, and while healthy. It has been found that this process is also critical during the development of mammals. It is a vital modulator of a number of disorders and diseases as well. The role of the pathway is better understood when you understand autophagy's involvement in both human development and diseases. The implication of this knowledge can be used to more effectively treat disease as well as support general health. While it is now understood how the process works from a general function and morphology, the pathway is intricate and the exact steps in the process are still being discovered.

Autophagy Mechanisms

Large molecules are broken down in cells through multiple catabolic pathways. One of the most notable pathways is the collaboration of ubiquitin, a small protein, with an additional cellular protein. After, this typically leads to more ubiquitin molecules to create a chain of polyubiquitin. This releases amino acids, using proteasome to mark the protein for degradation. Other, similar mechanisms for degradation exist with additional biological polymers. For example, this process exists for lipids and carbohydrates as well.

There are two reasons why autophagy is unique: first, it is able to select what and how much cargo it wants to carry, and, second, it is very flexible. It can encourage degradation for a substantial variety and number of substrates, allowing cells to rapidly and effectively recycle the materials used in basic cellular building. This is especially important in the face of nutrient deficiency. In addition, the pathway of autophagy is the single one able to degrade an entire organelle. It can do this in a targeted manner or at random. This crucial process balances the complicated setting for eukaryotic cells.

The process is very regulated, only releasing and increased when necessary. It is also tightly monitored so it can respond in a timely fashion. The TOR complex 1, or a cell's main metabolic sensor, is highly aware of how much amino acids and growth factors are present. It prevents autophagy when there is an abundance of these in the cell. When there are not enough of these present in the cell, the TOR complex 1 is turned "off," and autophagy is allowed to increase. While this is happening, additional molecular regulators keep an eye on cells for the levels of various nutrients, like glucose, or ATP energy. When the receptors sense that these items are low, they trigger autophagy.

Once autophagy begins, multiple proteins related to autophagy, called Atg, come together to create the phagophore and the next steps of autophagy. In the 1990s, the ATG genes of yeast were discovered. This discovery altered the course of autophagy research and the understanding of the process forever. Prior to this discovery, autophagy was just a generic description of the process. After this, science understood that the process is a major mechanism occurring at the molecular level. Autophagy's primary mechanism was further defined in a study using Saccharomyces cerevisiae, budding yeast that is genetically tractable. After this, more research in other organisms has followed. This spiral of discovery showed the world the conservative evolution in the function and nature of the machinery in autophagy in all living forms—from humans to yeast.

Scientists are fairly clear about the process of autophagy, but the puzzle is far from being completed. There are still many missing pieces to the overall picture of autophagy. For example, it still remains to be established by autophagosome's membrane donor. In addition, scientists still cannot determine precisely how regulations of the expansion of the phagophore are accomplished. It is not understood how frequent autophagosome is generated. Additional questions come up when scientists look at the various types of autophagy and its selectivity as well as the mystery of the triggering and regulation process. Human disease, healthy development and growth, and development of embryos have all been linked to the autophagy process; hence, uncovering more information about the process is vital for human homeostasis.

When Autophagy Goes Wrong

Cancer, neurodegenerative disorders, and infectious disease are pathologies all linked to the deregulation of the autophagy process. As more research is produced, it is becoming more evident that the relationship between disease and autophagy is vital to creating more effective therapies and interventions for some of the worst human diseases impacting our society today.

Yasuko Rikihisa of the College of Veterinary Medicine at Virginia Tech, first reported the induction of autophagy in 1984. The study produced showed that when incubated mammalian cells were infected with a tick-borne illness, rickettsiae, the cells triggered autophagosomes to be formed. Unfortunately, the understanding of this process on eukaryotic cells has just begun. Part of this process has shown to limit inflammation. Inflammation is critical to helping the body heal from infection or disease, but extended inflammation can cause tissue damage and other diseases. These preliminary findings suggest that in addition to monitoring the elimination of pathogens, it can also prevent unnecessary tissue degradation by limiting the presence of inflammation at the site.

At the Weill Cornell Medical College, J. Magarian Blander discovered that autophagy is vital to the stress response pathway of a cell when there is an infection present. The autophagy process is necessary for triggering the immune response after the stress is found in an infected cell. But at the Jan Lunemann's lab at the University of Zurich, it was discovered that it was not always helpful to modulate the immune system through autophagy. The process of autophagy may actually aggravate diseases like multiple sclerosis, or MS, which is an autoimmune disease impacting the central nervous system. Nerve degeneration and autoimmune disease is still an uncertain area for autophagy.

It is clear, however, that one of the main roles of autophagy is protection against several neurodegenerative disorders, like Parkinson's Disease and Huntington's Disease. One of the main culprits that lead to Huntington's disease—the mutant HTT, an aggregation-prone protein—is degraded through autophagy, according to the research published by David Rubinsztein and his colleagues at the Cambridge Institute for Medical Research. With regard to Parkinson's disease, reduction of mitophagy is a primary reason for pathogenesis. This is not surprising and the understanding that homeostasis of mitophagy is necessary for healthy neurological functioning.

Cancer is also connected to autophagy. The Levine Group discovered in 1999 that mice with only one autophagy-related gene, Becn-1, had more tumors. Research has shown that autophagy is critical in preventing tumor creation and also in stopping malignancy in present tumors. The generation and progression of tumors have several factors that respond to this dual role autophagy plays in the process. Tumors are prevented because autophagy suppresses the known stressors that cause tumor growth, such as mitochondrial dysfunction, metabolic disruption, and genomic instability. But once a tumor is created, the "playing field" changes dramatically. Growth and proliferation of a cell with a tumor have more metabolic demands than a healthy cell. But because of cancer, the vasculature cannot supply it with the necessary nutrients. This means the cell relies on upregulating autophagy to meet its growing needs. This means that inhibiting autophagy can actually help "starve" cancer cells. The challenge scientists face with this knowledge is the balance necessary for tumor starvation without also causing neurodegeneration and increasing the likelihood of infection. Because the process is not straightforward and autophagy is still being revealed, it is important the therapies using autophagy for cancer treatment are approached with extreme care.

The study of autophagy is still underway and a popular field for exploration. It is exciting is for science to explore because of the many benefits it provides to our bodies. It plays a critical role in our health and wellbeing. While some crucial and beneficial mechanics have been revealed over the last several decades, understanding of autophagy is still in its early stages. Things related to the initiation, progression, and regulation have provided the present understanding of autophagy, but there are still many questions that scientists are looking to answer. In fact, many would say there are still more questions than answers, especially regarding proteins related to autophagy. Therapeutic intervention, in particular, is looking into the role autophagy plays in the process of pathophysiology. It is interesting to recognize that a person's instinctual need to eat to stay alive extends beyond the need to consume food, but it includes the need to eat oneself, at least, on a cellular level.

Understand the Difference Between Psychological and Physical Hunger

Circadian clocks afford animals to predict daily events instead of ordinarily reacting to them. Also, the cells that create ghrelin possess circadian clocks that probably synchronize the expectation of food with metabolic cycles. In a nutshell, this means that eating a set of meals per day is trained and mastered behavior.

Most times we seem that we are hungry, we're not feeling true physiological or body hunger, rather what we're experiencing is psychological or head hunger. Immediately we notice this, then all it will take is to be disconnected from it until our system adapts to the fasting routine.

My Experience

In theory, fasting seems very easy. You could be thinking - yeah I will only avoid eating for some days and then continue with your meal afterward, but it goes beyond that. Personally, I have taken part in every type of fasting and failed several times. Every attempt I make looks pretty simple at the beginning. I used to be very excited concerning my latest plan that even the thought of eating never comes to my mind; I'd be so confident that I could bet on my success.

I'm committed at the starting of every fast that I would choose to stick with one. Meaning it's not until 20hrs plus that the interest of the fast starts to depreciate, and I begin to lose the motivating spirit to keep going. However, now I understand that what kept me quitting was that I thought I would reach the initial slump, which is unavoidable because everyone fasting goes through it as well. To me seems as if my brain is testing me to know if this is really what I desire.

It will be obvious to you when you hit the slumping state because, at that point, you'll be asking yourself whether you're doing the right thing, the mind will randomly remind you to eat something. But if you can be able to defeat that urge, you'll be empowered to continue your fast. That slump should be seen as a battle, in which you must fight and win to accomplish your goal. Make sure you're prepared for it and also expect it.

Fasting isn't an easy task, The beginning might be interesting to you, but it becomes tougher as time progresses, to the extent that you'll feel like giving up and eating anything in the cupboard or even buying a pizza to sustain the moment. AVOID DOING IT.

Follow this advice to succeed. Do yourself a favor and be sure to practice these tips before giving up.

- Always expect hunger
- Draft a plan detailing your strategy when you begin to feel the hunger

Take Tea or Coffee Without Adding Sugar

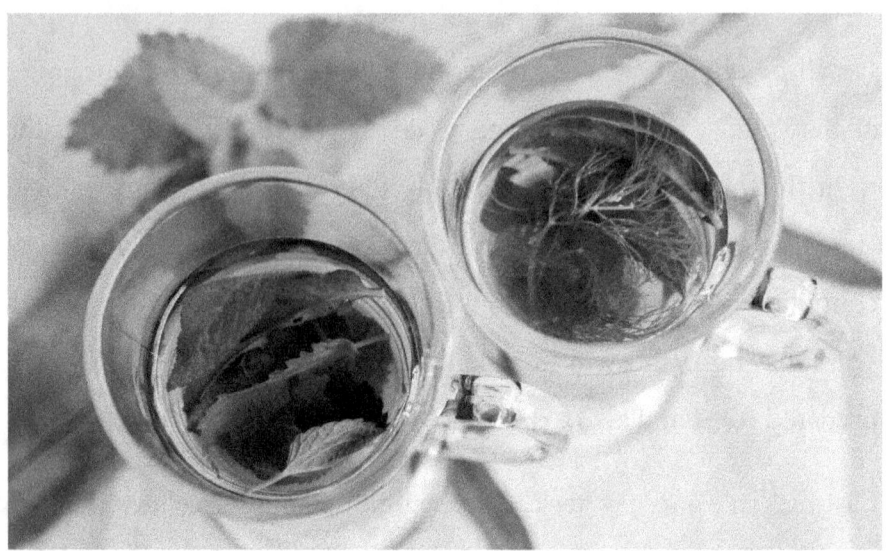

Everyone knows that caffeine provides you with energy, but not everyone knows it's a potent appetite suppressant. Coffee/tea can be used to stop the urge to eat for the whole day. Drinking hot tea or coffee can help in making a person feel as if he or she has eaten. Also, the truth that you're drinking something tasty makes it feel a lot like a meal.

Here's the question, should you use milk or not?

When your aim of fasting is to shed weight, then adding a small quantity of milk to your drink is healthy while those who are fasting for religious reasons or cleansing could brew their drink without adding milk.

If you prefer to be very strict, consume it black, although it doesn't make so much difference. You could add a dash of milk (not more than 6ml) and still be in a fasted state.

- Caffeine in tea/coffee represses your appetite
- Adding milk won't stop your fast

Ensure You're Drinking Plenty of Water

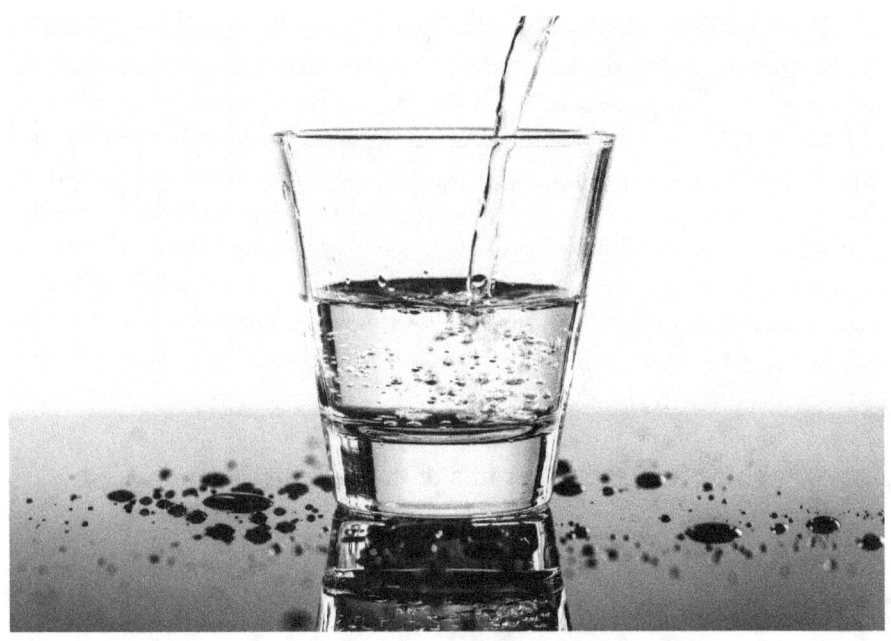

Thirst can appear like hunger. It might seem as if you're starving, but in the real sense, you're dehydrating. During fasting, a lot of water is removed from your body. Consume 2-3 liters of water daily when fasting. Lethargy and headaches are notable signs of dehydration, so when you experience these during fasting, drink more and more water. But if you aren't feeling the thirst to drink enough water, it could be that you've gotten to balance of salt-to-water in your blood. To solve this problem, add a small pinch of pink Himalayan salt into your water. It will also contribute to your electrolytes too.

Water is wonderful as it makes you feel fulfilled, but don't over consume it. Drinking massive amounts of water frequently will do more harm to you than good. The idea is to drink water whenever you feel hungry because consuming water unnecessarily will only make you urinate frequently and this flushes out your electrolytes that may cause flu-like symptoms. Make sure to stick with 2-3 liters and space out your durational consumption, and you'll be okay.

- Drink it when hunger comes knocking
- 2-3 liters every day
- Spread the water intake throughout the entire day

Go to Bed

It's baffling to note that a lot of people don't know that sleeping equals fasting as well.

The evening is the peak time that most people will break their fast, including me. I'll abide by it every day, and then when evening comes around, I give in and join my family during dinner. Whenever this happens, I see it as a failure in my part by writing off the week and starting anew on Monday of another week. The whole thing will want to repeat itself over and over again.

I have realized going to bed earlier would help me succeed that hard part, and waking up 8 hrs later it would've been the next morning. It's very hard to break your fast in the night if you follow this trick. Breaking your fast will make you feel bad the next day, rather than good, so try to sleep and see whether you'll still be hungry by morning.

It's advisable to begin your fast before going to bed, and using this strategy will make your first 8 hrs of fasting much easier and hunger-free.

- If you desire to give up when evening comes around, fight that urge off strongly
- Try to sleep whenever you're hungry at night

Remember that hunger comes in waves. It will pass.

Many people don't understand how long hunger takes because they're prompted to eat something whenever they get little feeling of hunger. They're always afraid of the word "hunger" and began to eat anytime their system churns with hunger. Those who are used to fasting know that if you endure a bit, the hunger will leave. Just put it in your mind you'll eat later because even feelings of hunger don't take more than 20 minutes or so, which starts to reduce as time passes.

Hunger is as a result of increased ghrelin. That is, ghrelin increases when you begin fasting, which leads to hunger. The increased levels of ghrelin don't remain permanent, meaning hunger reduces as fasting continues. During your weight loss journey ensure you also have this in mind. When the hiccups come around during that feeling of hunger remember to tell yourself: "This feeling of hunger in me will vanish soon" then moves on with your fasting.

- Hunger pangs only stay for 20 minutes before it starts to vanish
- Your hormone ghrelin causes the feeling of hunger
- The level of ghrelin reduces during ketosis

Distract Yourself

Human beings tend to mistake boredom for hunger. We tend to eat whenever we're bored because it keeps us busy. I was ignorant of how much eating food took out of my time during the day until I began to fast. I use to think that only the time spent on a meal is only the time we took to eat, but it was wrong. Thinking of what to consume at breakfast, lunch, dinner and what we'll eat during those times takes out a considerable amount of time spent because we spend much time thinking about it before eventually eating it.

It doesn't make sense when we start fasting, and our mind is still preoccupied with food. This happens because we have our normal day wired out of habit to be around food. So much so that even when you're not hungry, your system still triggers you to consume something as you keep thinking about it throughout the day.

How do you fight this anomaly during fasting? Try to distract yourself.

Try to pamper yourself. Personal care during fasting is my favorite strategy to kill time. Although fasting is difficult, take some time out to reward yourself. Immerse yourself in the tub with Epsom salts and read or listen to an interesting book. Go out and get a good haircut. Take a spa day. You're going through something incredibly difficult, and you deserve to be pampered.

Be organized. Organizing or cleaning around the house is another great distraction you could follow. For me, I always try to make lists of things during my non-fasting days that I'll do while fasting.

There are always little things we need to do around our home, office, and so on. They seem always to bother you but haven't made time for them. Now is your chance to take care of those bothersome errands. You could empty the messy closet that you've been using for years to be cleaned, clean and rearrange your storage cupboard, clean the dishes and wash your car, or delve into other chores. Some distractions that come with physical involvement can be very effective and also give you a light workout too.

Indulge Yourself. There's absolutely nothing embarrassing in engaging in unproductive activities to help you pass through a fast state because using few hours to play is better than giving up to achieve your desired result due to boredom. Watch videos on YouTube, watch your desired TV program, play games, and more.

I resort to checking my email, replying to Twitter or Facebook messages, whenever I feel bored and hungry. Normally, I would've stopped myself from doing these as it's unproductive, but I believe that it's better to be unproductive than to fail my fast because I know my health matters!

It's not difficult to realize when it's boredom that you're suffering from and not hunger. When you notice this, try to play around for some minutes to push through. Once the hunger vanishes, you can start your work again.

Go out for a walk. Most times, leaving the house or office is very helpful in keeping you going when you feel like giving up. You could decide to go to the store and buy some sparkling water, or tea, go and visit a friend. Even getting up to walk around the house or work with no aim in mind helps too.

When I reach the point that I'm doing this, I try to remember that my aim is my overall health and well-being. I imagine how happy I will be after achieving my goal and how people will feel after seeing me lose weight. Thinking of this while fresh air cools my frayed nerves keeps me inspired to move on with my fast.

Focus. By using your brain power effectively, your mind will automatically ignore thinking of food. Try to learn new things and put them into practice immediately like learning a new language or even a new hobby. Personally, I throw myself into a book or something that needs my full attention.

Nevertheless, the higher level of adrenaline and orexin in your system will help you to be up-and-doing, meaning your brain can take-in educative information easily and comfortably. Put it into practice, and you'll be surprised at how useful you can be with that extra time you're not worried over what to eat.

- Those times that you think you're hungry not knowing you're only bored
- Delve into your normal routine and get rid of boredom

Flee from Places Where You Can Smell or See Food

This reason made me break a lot of my fasts in the beginning. As I move on with my fasting confidently, thinking nothing will be able to stop me, I accidentally smell delicious food from somewhere. That very next moment I'd go for that meal and start eating, knowing I won't be happy with myself for the next 20 minutes. I suffered from this problem for quite a while, and I also know that it will happen again. I began to wonder the reason why I couldn't hold myself back since I knew it wasn't hunger, but I kept falling to that little test. So what was it?

We're programmed in a way that if we see or smell food, we start salivating to it. Immediately our digestive system opens for food intake, and our mouths began to water. Before we know it, our brain starts screaming at us to Eat! Eat!! Eat now!!!

It will take you a monk's discipline to resist eating food. Even if you don't, don't beat yourself up too much about it. The easiest and only way to avoid this is to stay away from hot food in those few days of your fast. As those days pass, you would be in ketosis and resisting won't be challenging any longer.

If you're the type that cooks for other people like yourself, make them understand that you're in your fasting days and can't cook for those periods. If that isn't possible, you could buy takeout food or schedule preparing a meal for them during your non-fasting days.

- Being close to food will make your body want to eat
- Resisting the urge to eat is incredibly difficult when your brain is pushing you to eat something

Meditate

You can remove yourself from feelings of hunger by practicing meditation. Push yourself far away from the urge to eat until that cravings disappear.

One other best idea to eliminate hunger or craving for food is to shift your focus. Whether you're fasting or not, meditation helps greatly to rid your head-space, but together with fasting, meditation and fasting enhance and synergize each other.

- You're free to meditate at any point in time
- For beginners, it's healthy to practice guided meditation

Remember Why You Started

Always remember that you engaged in fasting for a purpose, and not for the sake that you don't feel like eating. Try to write the reasons that made you go into fasting, daily. What's that thing you want to change by fasting? Are you fasting for personal reasons? And why?

Try to write down the reasons you're fasting after doing it today. Do it tomorrow as well, because most people easily forget their reasons for doing something. Make it a habit of reminding yourself daily by writing it down as many times as possible so that it will be imprinted in your brain.

From now on anytime your memory tells you to eat it will immediately ring in your head that you're fasting.

- So write those reasons down so you'll know them by heart
- Don't forget that it's only you who can personally end the fast

Habit Changes

Anyone who fasts to lose weight and yet doesn't make any habit/diet changes will gradually recover all the weight used up during the fasting period

If your goal for doing a water fast is to lose weight, ensure your first focus is to change your eating habits, then gradually proceed to water fasting via the previously explained methods. Upon returning to your usual self, stick to your changed diet habit.

Old habits vs. New habits – begins with:

- Staying away from animal products: All dairy products, eggs, and meat. You'll shed so much weight by doing this, and it'll make you look and feel a lot better.

- Along with every meal, eat a big serving of green leafy salad.

- Include one freshly extracted vegetable juice in your everyday routine.

- Also, in your everyday meal plan, include activated charcoal and alkaline water in your diet.

- Engage in one short water fast every week, or intermittent water fast every month, or 3-day extended water fast every three months.

Following these steps will help you ensure success in stopping the old habits and keeping the new habits.

CHAPTER 3: THE BENEFITS OF AUTOPHAGY

1. **It enhances the body's fitness.** Fasting helps the body to burn fats, and as such, the body will feel lighter and such individual can be said to be fit.

2. **Promotes greater satiety.** Your adipocytes produce various hormones (acting as an endocrine organ), such as your leptin which regulates the way you feel. When you fast; however, you burn most of these stored fatty tissues, your leptin levels drop automatically (creating a leptin-deficient environment). Hence, whenever the little amount of leptin is produced, the effect is heightened, and your body becomes more responsive to leptin thereby modulating how you feel after a meal.

3. **Enhanced metabolism.** Leptin is also known as the (satiety hormone) also stimulate the production of thyroid hormones. Thus, enhanced leptin responsiveness will directly increase the rate of metabolism.

4. **Facilitates fat loss and ketosis.** Fat-loss or ketosis can be accomplished either by eating a Ketogenic Diet or by fasting. A Ketogenic Diet helps to burn out stored fat which is harmful rather than helpful to the body

organs such as the liver, the kidneys, and the blood vessels.

5. **Enhances insulin sensitivity:** When you fast, the body secretes a lesser amount of insulin which in turn increases insulin sensitivity.

6. **Boosts cardiovascular health:** Fasting is recommended for those who wish to improve their cardiovascular function and have normal blood pressure.

7. **Reduced blood pressure.** Most people experience lower BP while fasting. This effect could be as a result of lower salt consumption and increased salt loss through urine.

8. **Lower blood sugar.** The blood sugar could drop as much as over 30 percent within a few days of fasting, and if care is not taken, the person could become hyperglycemic.

9. **Decreases blood triglycerides.** The triglycerides content of the blood drops low while an individual is fasting which helps to increase the blood flow within the blood vessels which could have been narrowed by fat components.

10. **Better heart condition.** Fasting has been found to help reduce the accumulation of free radicals within the body. Free radicals are harmful to the muscles of the heart.

11. **Could slow the rate of aging and prolong your lifespan.** There have been positive results obtained from animal studies to prove that fasting could prolong lifespan. Also, when the blood is cleaned regularly, it slows down the process of aging and improves the health of an individual.

12. **Suppresses inflammation.** Although several factors cause inflammation, an unhealthy diet could lead to increased production of free radicals which in turn could cause inflammation. Food items such as alcohol, refined food items, fried foods, etc. are all sources of free radicals.

13. **Reduces the effects of Oxidative Stress.** When the rate at which free radicals are produced is higher than the rate at which it is eliminated, it accumulates in the body thereby causing oxidative stress which is damaging to the cells of the body.

14. **Enhances cellular recycling process.** Senescent cells accumulate in our body as we age. But when we fast,

the body activates the process of self-digestion, and along the line, malignant cells are also destroyed.

15. **Growth regulation.** It has been found that insulin-like growth factor 1 (IGF-1) could lead to the proliferation of cancer. But fasting suppresses the production of IGF-1.

16. **Protects the brain.** Research works carried out on the function of the brain and aging have revealed one could age gracefully by fasting regularly.

17. **Promotes a healthy stress response.** Moderate stress is beneficial to the brain especially when it is infrequent, and fasting can induce such stress. Moderate stress triggers a series of activities that are protective to the brain cells (neurons).

18. **Promotes recovery from an injury.** Though the mechanism is not fully understood, research from animal models has shown that intermittent fasting helps the healing process.

19. **Supports healthier skin collagen production.** Your skin is a reflection of your diet. Accumulation of glucose can compromise the structure of the collagen, but fasting can help you overcome this challenge and give your skin that glow.

Side Effects of Fasting

Everyone fasts for various reasons such as: to lose weight, for a religious purpose, for healthy living and the list go on. A fast could either be mild or strict (ranging from liquid only such as juice, tea, coffee and the likes to no food, no fluid). Although fasting comes with a lot of benefits, it also has its associated downsides, which could either be short term or long term. These effects vary from one individual to another.

Poor weight management. Many people tend to crave for and consume more calories after a long period of fasting, which will inevitably counteract all the progress, made by fasting.

Short-term downsides. Fasting could have several adverse effects such: dizziness, headaches, outbursts, weakness, low blood pressure, gouts/gall stones among others.

Long-Term downsides. Continuous prolonged fasting could weaken the immune system and affect vital organs such as the kidneys and the liver. When an individual abstains from food over a long period, he becomes malnourished and could lead to an untimely death after the entire energy store of the body has been exhausted.

Dry Fast. Dry fasting is the most dangerous form of fasting in which an individual abstains from food and fluids. It could even lead to death if other underlying factors such as exertions, heat and the likes set in.

Water Fasting. There is a high tendency of losing the wrong type of weight while performing this form of fasting. This is because this form of fasting only allows the intake of water but restrict one from taking in calories. Although an individual could lose up to 0.9kg (2 pounds) 24-72 hours of water fasting, sadly, such weight loss can be a loss of carbohydrates, muscle mass and even water.

Possible dehydration. As funny as it may sound, water fasting could still cause dehydration because about 20-30 percent of our daily water intake comes from the food we eat. Thus, if we consume the same amount of water as we do on average days, we could experience some symptoms of dehydration such as light-headedness, dizziness, constipation, headaches, weakness, nausea, etc. To prevent such unwanted side effects, you may need to increase your water consumption.

Possibility of experiencing Orthostatic Hypotension. This type of hypotension is usually common among those whose fast. You might have experienced something similar when you get up suddenly, and then you feel dizzy or lightheaded. A sudden drop in the blood pressure causes that feeling, and such ones are prone to fainting. If you think you are experiencing orthostatic hypotension, then it means your body is not compatible with water fasting.

Water fasting could worsen a medical condition: Those with certain medical conditions should avoid water fasting as it could worsen such conditions:

- **Gout**: Gout is caused by an accumulation of Uric acid in the joints, and water fasting could increase its production.

- **Diabetes**: In Type I and type II diabetes, fasting could aggravate the side effect of diabetes.

- **Chronic kidney disease**: Those with chronic kidney condition should avoid water fast as it may worsen such condition.

- **Eating disorders**: Bulimia nervosa could be enhanced by fasting. There is more than sufficient evidence to back this up.

- **Heartburn:** Heartburn may be induced by fasting as the body will keep producing gastric acid which helps the digestion process.

Precautions to Take When Fasting

Fasting has a lot of advantages. However, fasting is not meant for everyone. To better understand the theory of fasting, let us compare Fasting to a tool (such as an arrow) which can either be used properly or misused. Holding to that, we will use the archery metaphor to explain the effective use and the misuse of fasting/autophagy. A hunter could have different sizes and tips of arrows in his quiver. When he finds an antelope, he will use a sharp wooden arrow, but when faced by a lion or bear, he would go for something stronger: probably an arrow with metallic tips. The point is don't use the wrong method for the right purpose.

Who should avoid fasting

Pregnant and breastfeeding mothers. Whether you have a child you're breastfeeding or one who is still in your uterus, you need all the calories you can get; both the mother and the infant need to be fed well to stay nourished and healthy.

Underaged students and those below 18 should avoid Fasting. Children under the age of 18 are still growing and need all the vital nutrients and minerals to have healthy growth and development.

Those that is underweight and/or malnourished. If you find it difficult to tell whether you are malnourished or not, you could ask your physician or a trusted friend. Those having an eating disorder such as bulimia are included in this category.

Individuals who have Type-2 Diabetes. Fasting has been used over the years as a means of reversing the effect of Type-2 diabetes. However, you still need to consult your physician before beginning a fast.

Who needs to be cautious?

Another group of individuals who also need to be cautious is those with occasional gastroesophageal reflux disease (GERD). Those who fall into this category need to check with their physician as well if they wish to fast and must be closely monitored.

There are solid pieces of evidence to prove that GERD could be aggravated by fasting and the symptoms could become worsened. This possible worsening is because during fasting, the stomach will be devoid of food and there will be nothing which the gastric juice would digest.

Individuals on medications need to be cautious while fasting as the fasting periods could overlap when such drugs would be taken especially those medications that would require you to eat before using them.

In addition, those on cancer therapy and other medical treatment must be cautious and should have an in-depth discussion with their physician before fasting.

CHAPTER 4: HOW AUTOPHAGY MAY IMPROVE THE QUALITY AND LENGTH OF YOUR LIFE

Some things are dependent on one another such as water fasting, the ketogenic lifestyle, and autophagy. One of the more popular methods of activating autophagy is by undergoing a ketogenic diet.

Before proceeding, it is essential to note that the Ketogenic Diet does not enhance your capability to go without eating- every machine requires an energy source. The mechanism by which keto works is by providing your body with a method of using a more persistent energy source obtained from heavy fats instead of carbohydrates. Normally, people who are not used to the Ketogenic Diet experience hunger pangs when they do not eat snacks for a few hours. These hanger pangs can be regularly seen in people that are dependent on quickly depleted carbs. If you already have previously adapted to keto, you should be able to function without food for days and without any need to eat.

Fasting lowers the level of insulin and blood sugar which promotes the secretion of hormones that deplete fats, like adrenaline and glucagon. This then supports the degradation of fats known as triglyceride reserves in adipose tissue. Eventually, when triglycerides are transported to the liver, they are used as a source of fuel or to generate ketone bodies. Once your ketone levels become about 7-8 mmol/L that's when you know your body has begun ketosis.[29]

As a result of reduced carbohydrate intake, the ketogenic diet results in a decrease in the levels of insulin and glucose. Contrary to fasting, some amount of protein and foods rich in fats are permitted. Unlike glucose, fats and proteins do not significantly affect the levels of blood glucose.

Contrarily, fat does not have this effect, eating a diet rich in fat, but low in protein and carbs divert your energy source to ketone bodies and imitates a natural, fasted condition. This means that by being in a ketotic state, you would be stimulating autophagy.[30]

Furthermore, lowering your intake of protein and carbohydrates, in turn, lowers the number of poisonous substances that are absorbed by your body, so there is just a little toxin for your body to eliminate, making autophagy even more fully effective.

This is probably why people that engage in the keto diet start feeling like an improved version of themselves. Their bodies are eliminating toxins, and there is an upgrade in their health.

One of the main proponents of the ketogenic diet is water fasting because digesting even the healthiest meals uses energy and can stress the body eventually. Water fasting helps the body to rest and permits recycling of excess energy.

Additionally, the body enters into a ketotic state more rapidly if you are on a water fast. Water fasting creates extended, more efficient periods of ketosis. Also, a more intense restoration at cellular levels is observed while on a water fast.

Even though this is similar to what happens on a Ketogenic Diet, but water fasting makes the process faster with the additional advantages we have discussed previously.

The type of fat used to generate ketones is one other difference between water fasting and a keto diet. Fat reservoirs are the source of fat when you are on a fast. However, the fat in keto is gotten from the high-fat meals you are consuming. The quantity of calories gotten from your dietary fat determines if a ketogenic diet would result in weight loss.

Start Fasting Gradually

It might be challenging to undergo a water fast, but your body starts to adapt to the recent changes eventually. Within the first three days, you might be tempted to stop. The smell of food excites you, and you will start to imagine all the foods you would get to eat after breaking your fast. By day three, ketosis is complete, and you will start to feel dizzy if you get up too fast, have intense headaches, and sleep disturbances.

After two weeks, you would no longer feel the intense headaches and hunger pangs. You might still feel dizzy and very cold because the levels of your blood pressure are still lower than normal. By then you can easily cook family meals without temptations, and you would begin to detest the smell of sugary snacks and unhealthy foods.

In comparison to the first two weeks, the third week should be easier because this is because the body is adapting to the recent changes and you have eliminated the majority of the toxins in your body lowering flu-like and discomforting after effects.

Begin with a small fast. How many hours can you go without food? Three hours? Six hours? Begin with that and gradually add one hour every day.

Remember: Before you start running – learn to walk first.

Most people make the common error of starting directly with 24-hour fasts when they are used to 3-6 meals each day together with snacks. In some cases, it is possible to attempt this, but it might begin to feel like torture and starvation.

Eating the Right Foods

On fasting days, eat a little bit of food. Generally, fasting entails partially or completely going without food or drinks for a certain period.

Though it is possible to exclude food completely on fasting days, a few fasting strategies such as the 5:2 diet permits you to eat about 25% of your calorie needs in one day.[31]

If you are thinking of starting a fast, limit your caloric intake to enable yourself to eat small quantities during your fasting days. Limiting your intake can be healthier than engaging in a complete fast when you're starting as a beginner.

This method might help to lower the risks of fasting like experiencing hunger, inability to concentrate or light-headedness.

Because you do not feel really hungry, it might also make it easier to continue with the fast.[32]

Ensure Adequate Hydration. It is important to drink sufficient amounts of liquid while on a fast because thirst, fatigue, headaches, and dry mouths can be caused by mild dehydration.

Many health experts advise people to use the 8 by 8 rule- 8 glasses that are 8 oz. in size (less than 2 liters) of liquid each day- to ensure adequate hydration.

Although this might be enough, the quantity of liquid you need depends on you as an individual. It is very easy to become dehydrated while fasting because 20-30% of the fluid required by your body comes from food.

While fasting, a lot of people try to drink 2-3 liters (8.5-13 cups) of water throughout the day. But, thirst should guide you on when it is time to drink additional water, follow the instructions that your body is telling. Only you know when too much water is too much.

Eat Plenty of Protein. For most people, fasting is a form of weight loss although you have to remember that a reduction in caloric intake will make you lose not just fat but muscle as well.

One method of reducing the risk of losing muscle while on a fast is to make sure that you are consuming sufficient amount of proteins on the days that you are allowed to eat food.[33]

Also, adding protein to the small-sized meals on your fast days can help suppress your hunger and provide other beneficial effects.

Some researchers propose that getting 30% of your calories by eating protein can significantly suppress your appetite.[34]

Because of this, some bad after effects of fasting can be reduced by consuming some form of good protein.

Avoid ending your Fasts With large Meals. After fasting for a while, the thought of ending your fast with a large meal can be enticing but ending you fast with a large meal can make you weak and bloated. Also, if you desire to lose weight, large meals might impede your fasting objectives by impeding or stopping your weight loss process.

Eating too many calories after a fast lowers your caloric deficit because your total caloric intake affects your health, so the most effective way of ending a fast is to keep eating normally and continue with your usual eating schedule

Exercise while fasting. Before starting any workout routine, consult your doctor, especially when you are fasting. Your doctor knows your medical history and can specifically advise you on what to do. Also, tell your doctor about your wish to fast and your workout routine, so your doctor would know if this is suitable or unsafe.

Stop the fast and workout if you experience any discomfort or pain when exercising, or the aftereffects of a fast, and you are advised to call your doctor instantly. Your doctor would decide if your heart could cope with exercises when you are on a fast.

How does it feel to workout while fasting? This is determined by many factors, ranging from the fasting approach you use to the response of your body has to the fast. Following your body's directions is pertinent. If fasting makes you too tired to exercise, solve your nutrition issues first, then you can exercise later.

Although safety should be your priority, a number of exercise routines can enhance fasting.

Schedule your meals around your exercises. Cardio can be done on an empty stomach. You are allowed to go on a jog or register for that early morning spin session. However, it is vital to select the right foods before you attempt any form of cardio.

Since you know you would be working out, you should carefully select what to eat on the previous day as determined by how hard you would be exercising. For instance, you may want to increase your glycogen reserves by eating complex carbohydrates for dinner, the previous night so that you would be provided with easily accessible energy for your cardio exercise. It is inadvisable to do cardio when your stomach is full because the muscle's abrupt demand for blood diverts the important blood required for nutrient digestion and absorption. The best thing is to make plans beforehand to ensure that your nutrition provides the nutrients for your intense exercise, even though you would be exercising the following morning.

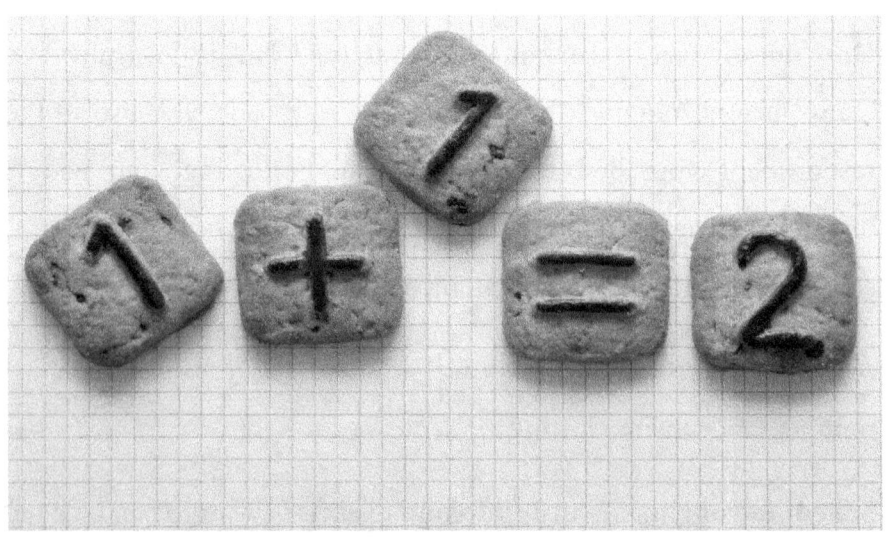

Exercise Suggestions For You

Choose less stressful exercises. While on a fast, a simple exercise might be very helpful because it makes sure that your body does not convert protein to an energy source.

While fasting, your body is dependent on energy reserved in the form of glycogen (this is the form in which glucose is stored by your body) If it has been a while since you last ate, your glycogen reserved might have been depleted, and this would drive your body to use protein as a source of energy.

- Rather than working out by running, walk. Moderate walks are a less stressful way of increasing your heart rate.

- Engage in Tai Chi or light yoga. Gradual, precise movements stabilize and enhance your body, and this old approach is a popular way of clearing and soothing the mind.

- Engage in light yard chores or gardening. Gardening needs you to lift, bend or move in other ways. Yard work and gardening are both excellent activities that mimic exercise.

However the intense exercise may be, the moment you start to feel dizzy or weak, stop the exercise instantly. You might have to drink water and eat a small portion of food to bring your energy level back up.

The great thing is that engaging in less stressful workouts while fasting makes the body to start using fat as a source of energy. For people that are trying to lose weight, this is very beneficial.

Make sure your workout routine is practical. Rather than walking, you might feel like running, or you might feel that you can cope with lifting heavy weights. However, fasting alters the normal limits of your body.

If your fast is for a religious purpose, or a medical reason, make plans to include less stressful workouts that you can easily do. You can continue with your regular workout routine as soon as your fast has ended.

If your fast extends from dusk to dawn, you have to stay away from working out during those periods and make sure to workout at a time that is close to your eating periods in the morning or evening.

If the purpose of your fast is to lose weight or other health reasons, you have to include exercises with caution. Take care to do less stressful workouts on your fasting days, and engage in rigorous exercises on days that you eat extra calories.

When to Stop Working Out During Fasting. When fasting or working out, the most important thing to do is what your body is telling you because there is a large risk of reduction in the levels of your blood glucose. So if you have never done this before, do not register for a rigorous session that might involve maximum exertion of your heart. Do not overdo it. Overdoing it might make you feel light-headed or even lose consciousness due to a quick reduction in the levels of your blood glucose, and it is a scary situation when that happens.

A little bit of planning would be very beneficial. The most vital factor to consider while on an extended or intermittent fast is what your breakfast looks like and how it works well with your workout routine. It is vital to consume healthy fats, protein, organic fibers, and complex carbs during the eating period to sustain a healthy fast.

So, that's it. Rigorous, or less rigorous exercises, make sure to make suitable plans for your meals. Remember, the most important thing is to listen to your body. Do not engage in rigorous workouts if it's telling you not to do them. Throughout the fast, there will be a variation in your energy levels, from experiencing weakness and tiredness to experiencing energy bursts. Regardless of how energetic you feel, do not stress yourself. Rather, engage in calm, soothing yoga. Yoga is a gentle way of stretching out your muscles and engaging in mild exercises.

For some people, light stretches and yoga might be easy, and for others, it might be too rigorous. Do what makes you feel good and go from there.

The Significance of Sleep While Fasting

During water fasting, sleep is the next crucial thing after water intake. While sleeping, the body undergoes repair, restoration, detoxification, and metabolism. It also begins a growth phase where it stores up energy and the cells begin to grow. You're at an optimal state after a satisfactory 7-8 hours of sleep during fasting, and the rate of tissue renewal is increased while sleeping as opposed to being in an active state. Both sleep and fasting should complement each other to attain a better healthy body overall; therefore, a great advantage of fasting is its positive effect on sleep. Although during the fast, you may find it difficult to sleep as a result of the earlier energy surge, there will be a significant positive change in the pattern of sleep because of the regulation carried out by the body to bring back normalcy.

Professional GuidanceDuring Water-Fasting

With proper medical supervision and adequate guidance, water fasting is an efficient and harmless way of assisting the body in self-restoration. However, like any other things that affect the body, there are some associated risks. For anyone that is considering undergoing a therapeutic fast, my advice would be to do this under the guidance of a certified IAHP expert who is trained in the process. The International Association of Hygienic Physicians consists of primary care doctors that are experts at supervising therapeutic fasts. Every approved member is a licensed osteopath, medical doctor or chiropractor, that has finalized at least a 6-month residency program at an authorized institution that is specialized in therapeutic fasts. Unlike in the past, fasting is now easily accessible due to the increase in the number of licensed professionals

Advantages of fasting under professional guidance. Maximum health is sustained when the body has adequate health requirements such as proper environment, psychology, and diet. If any of these requirements are inadequate, it affects your health. Most times, therapeutic fasting is an incredibly effective way of health recovery since it enables the body to produce an exceptional response to healing.

No other form of fasting can mimic the benefits of this way of fasting. Fasting, in a busy, noisy, or unsupportive surrounding will deprive the body of the chance to optimize the processes of self-restoration. Total rest is pertinent to optimize the beneficial effects of therapeutic fasting. Drinking juices exclusively or eating particular foods are essential as well. There are tremendous benefits both health and physiologically-wise when you consume these foods. However, this does not imply that the elimination diet, otherwise known as juice diet, is better than a straight water fast.

How A Chiropractor Will Help With The Fasting Process

Certain specialists in the health care sector concentrate on recognizing, and treating diseases that affect the junction between muscles and nerves, and they are very particular about curing these diseases by molding and sometimes, even altering the spinal cord. These specialists are called Chiropractors.

Chiropractors educate their patients on how to care for themselves by ergonomics, exercising, making user-friendly systems and other remedies to relieve back pain. Their main aim is to lessen the pain felt by patients and to increase their performance.

They believe that periodic fasting purges the body of harmful substances and causes the body to perform optimally.

There are certain criteria chiropractors take heed of during a fast;

First on the list of criteria is preventing death. Chiropractors expect side effects of fasting such as irritability, skin rashes, foul taste in the mouth, headaches, nausea and vomiting, unusual discharges from mucous membranes, postural hypertension and low back pain in the initial stage of fasting as a result of referral activity from kidney changes.

These professionals know that their patients undergo characteristic restorative crisis whereby persistent illnesses develop into short term illnesses and that it can be very distressing. Thus, their responsibility is to detect the boy's attempt to recover through a short term illness.

They are very mindful of carrying out the proper clinical supervision of their patients, after which they monitor the reaction of the body to the fast to determine the extent and severity of the therapy. To a great length, chiropractors monitor patient's activities like the food they eat, the time they sleep, and even as far as how susceptible they are to levels of stress.

Chiropractors can guarantee a risk-free experience, influencing the slightest reaction to water fasting (including hydration), as a result of the control they have over the patient's activities.

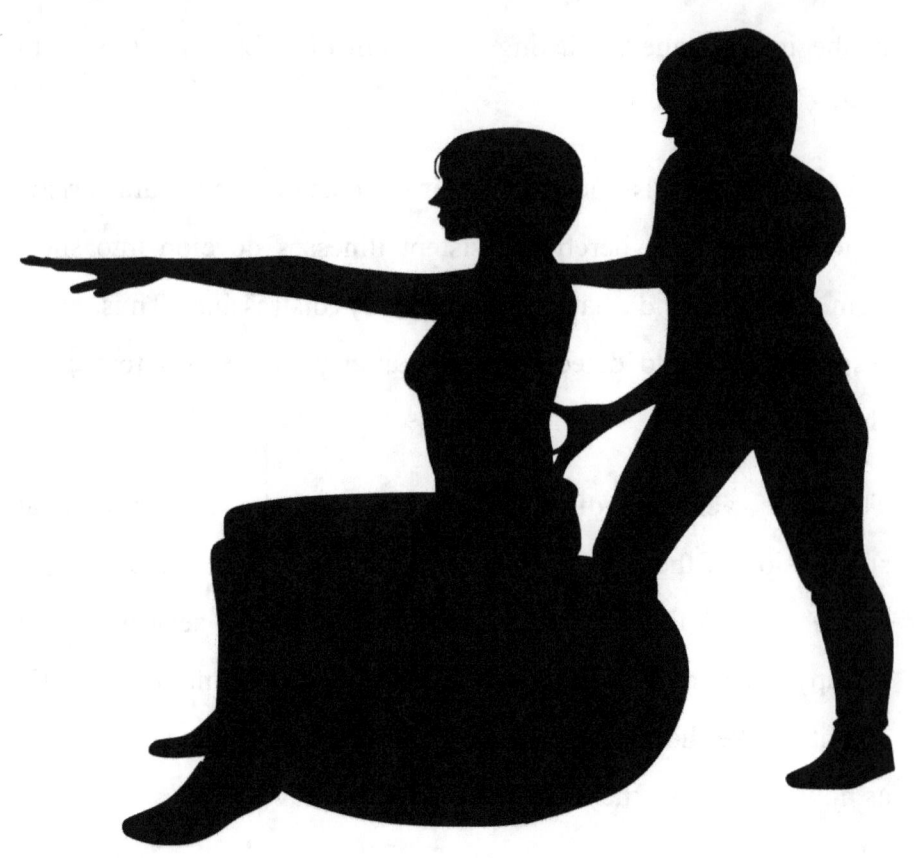

CHAPTER 5: REGULATION OF INFLAMMATION AND IMPROVED MUSCLE PERFORMANCE BY AUTOPHAGY

It is the preservation of life when the body is working to fight off something in times of stress or even starvation. This microscopic performance activates to repair the cells and any damage that could be caused by illness and inflammation. This process can also deplete or starve unwanted intruders from the vital nutrients they need to survive, allowing for their death and renewal.

The benefits of autophagy are limitless and can change your body function deep down on the cellular level. Some benefits are:

- **Promotion of a longer, healthier life through cell regeneration**
- **Helps in weight loss by encouraging healthier metabolism**—Autophagy can help clean and restore the toxic accumulation in the mitochondria, the energy makers of the cell. This is where fat gets burned and Adenosine Triphosphate (ATP) is produced. ATP is the compound that provides certain cellular energy, specifically muscle contraction. Autophagy allows for greater efficiency to boost metabolism and energy stores.

- **Risks of neurodegenerative disease are decreased**—Diseases in the brain take a long time to occur and happen over time with the buildup of misfolded, old, or dysfunctional proteins in or around the brain cells. The chemical compounds linked to the cause of Parkinson's disease, synuclein, is removed through autophagy. Studies suggest that the same may be true in cases of Alzheimer's, removing the compound amyloid from the brain that is known to be associated with this disease. Another neurodegenerative disease is dementia caused by diabetes. Chronic insulin resistance disallows autophagy from occurring so no clean up can occur within the cell, leaving them in a toxic wasteland of malfunction.
- **Regulation of inflammation**—Autophagy allows inflammation when it is needed to fight off invaders, yet also reduces inflammation when it is the chronic response to over-triggered signals to the cells and the body.
- **Helps fight infectious disease**
- **Improves muscle performance**—Muscles undergo stress during exercise. Microscopic tearing in the fibers of muscles occurs during strenuous activity. The muscle fibers, also made of specific kinds of cells, are

repaired through the process of autophagy. Over time, as you build muscle, it will reduce the amount of energy needed to utilize the muscle in general.

- **Prevents the onset of cancer**—Though research is still being done to understand the effects of autophagy on various kinds of cancer, studies have indicated that it can help to prevent cancer from forming. Scientists who have studied the impact of impaired autophagic response in mice see an up-rise of cancer in the mice. To perform the study, the mice involved had their autophagic response mechanism cut off from fully functioning. The result was cancer. The question is, can it work as a treatment for cancer, instead of just preventing it through autophagy? How would inducing autophagy impact other treatments? More research must be done to understand the impact of induced autophagy in pre-existing cancer treatments like chemotherapy, but it may be that it could have a greater benefit than chemo which can be incredibly damaging to the body if applied long term.
- **Improvement in digestive health**—Autophagy is activated through fasting for short periods intermittently. The break from calorie intake and digestion alone can help your digestive system immensely; everyone needs a break now and then.

More to that, while your body is resting from needing to digest, the cells that make up your digestive system and all other systems in your body will be activated to perform autophagy because of the fast, leading to a purification of the cells.

- **Improves the health of the skin**—Damage from sun exposure, toxins in the air, changes in temperature, acute ailments like bruises, scrapes, punctures, and burns may all benefit from the autophagic performance. While you may be constantly replacing cells, autophagy keeps the cells fresh and renewed, giving a glow to the skin.

- **Minimizes cell death or apoptosis**—With autophagy functioning, the cells are constantly being cleaned and rejuvenated; without it, the cells are piling up with waste and eventually struggle to perform well, leading to a programmed death of the cell. When that happens, the cell leaves behind trash that needs to be taken out, and if the cell itself is dead, autophagy won't occur because the process occurs inside the cell. The body will have to trigger an inflammatory response to clean up the cell death aftermath.

- **Improved cognition, memory, and brain function**—Autophagy enhances neuroplasticity, the brain's ability to form and reorganize synaptic connections. There is an increase in cognitive ability through the increase of mitochondria. When your brain cells can function well, so can your whole brain.

- **Regulation of hormones, which allows for overall body high performance and function.**
- **Improves cardiovascular health**—Autophagy works to clean toxins and biowaste from the cells of the heart muscle, which is constantly pumping blood through your whole body. Aiding in the general renewal of these cells brings about a better functioning heart.

The list goes on, and discoveries about the effects of autophagy on the health of the body continue to demonstrate the beneficial impact of the autophagic performance. When you create opportunities to enhance and promote autophagy, you are enhancing and promoting the health of every cell in your body.

Risks and Cautions of Performance Autophagy

Before you move ahead and begin the process of activating autophagy, it is important to be aware of cautions and risks. To have the best benefit from creating this healing response, you need to plan ahead and be informed about how to do it properly so that you don't cause yourself harm.

There are three main ways that you will learn to activate autophagy in this book: exercise, ketosis, and fasting. When covering the risks, you will understand what can happen or potentially go wrong while using these methods to activate autophagy. Bear in mind that if you are suffering from any severe medical issues, chronic illness, or disease, then it is always a good idea to consult a doctor before beginning this process.

This chapter will briefly cover some of the risks and precautions in initiating autophagy so that you can be prepared to plan your experience well. The next chapters in the book will go into greater detail about each method of activating autophagy.

Some risks and precautions:

- **Losing the wrong kind of weight**—If you lose muscle instead of fat, you are losing the wrong kind of weight. If you don't need to lose a lot of fat through diet, or fasting, then you have to ensure that you consume enough fat prior to fasting. Your body must be prepared to enter a period without calorie intake, and if you have no fat to burn, then you may find yourself losing some muscle. This is not usually the case if you are fasting properly, preparing in advance, and giving your body time to rest while you are on the fast. Some people will try to do intense exercise on a fast to create an even greater increase in the autophagic response.

This is when your body will start to turn to the protein of your body for energy. Make sure you are approaching fasting to induce autophagy healthily.

- **Dehydration**—During an intermittent water fast, you may run the risk of dehydration. Fasting is taking a break from food and food contains a percentage of your daily water intake. You will need to make sure you are drinking the right amount of water to stay hydrated. On the other hand, drinking too much water can drown the cells, and drinking too much, too fast can lead to hyponatremia which is the loss of sodium in the body. Loss of salt in your body can lead to an extreme drop in blood pressure. Drop in sodium levels due to excess water will cause fluid shifts from outside to inside the cell. The swell causes pressure in the skull which can lead to headache, nausea, and vomiting. Severe cases of decreased blood pressure can lead to confusion, problems breathing, sleepiness, confused state, weakened muscles, and cramping.
- **Urge to overeat after fasting**—Returning to food after a fast must be done slowly, in steps. When you are not healthily performing a fast, you may be inclined to overeat following the fasting period. If done regularly, this can have a detrimental impact on the body, causing shock to your system.

- **Extreme fasting can lead to starvation and eventually death**
- **If you fast for too long your body will start to eat itself**—If you are performing a fast for an extreme length of time without any calories, or supplements, your body will start to eat muscle, including cardiovascular muscle and also cells like brain cells. This can be avoided by choosing the right length of time for your fast, the right fast for your needs, and the right mineral and vitamin supplement to aid the process and prevent muscle loss. There is an important window of benefit for creating autophagy in a fast—between activation and the point where your body stops burning fat and starts eating muscle.
- **Loss of vitamins and minerals from food can cause health problems**—It is important to allow a mineral supplement. Since there are no calories in many supplements, you will not be breaking the fast, although some vitamins can cause discomfort in the stomach if not taken with food, so finding the right vitamins is important for fasting comfort.
- **Less serious, but important precautions and risks is the effect on mood**—Irritability, moodiness, highs and lows, energy depletion, low blood pressure, and dizziness.

- **Improper fasting can raise stress hormone levels-** If you are not engaging in fasting properly, you may encounter the issue of increased stress hormones in the body which isn't good for long periods and can be very damaging to many systems.
- **Fast detoxifying can impact your health**—The rate of detox when fasting is rapid. Toxins held in your body fat for long periods will release in your bloodstream as your body burns fat for calorie consumption. Too many toxins in the bloodstream can feel terrible and lead to nausea, sickness, and a general unwell feeling.
- **A fasting high can impact your cognitive ability**—Sometimes during a fast, you may experience fasting high, a feeling of euphoria as your body shifts and heals. Sometimes, this mental state can make it challenging for you to reasonably listen to your body, making sure you are not overdoing it.

A majority of the risks and precautions can be easily avoided if you approach autophagic performance with knowledge and preparation. Because the benefits of autophagy are so powerful, it is worth experiencing. With the right diet, exercise, fasting, and rest, you can healthfully activate autophagy safely and beneficially.

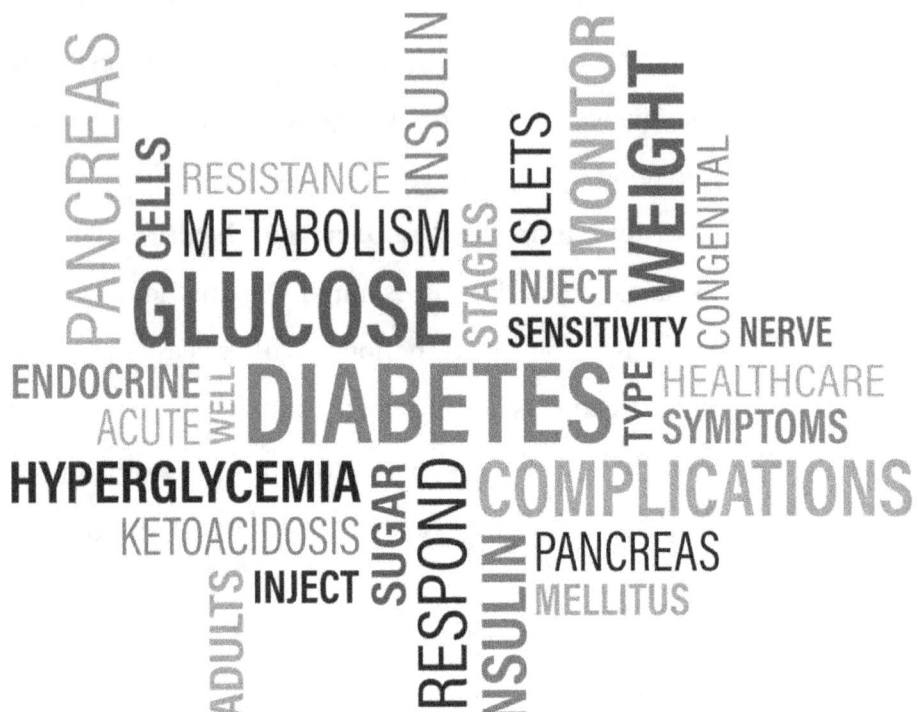

CHAPTER 6: AUTOPHAGY IMPROVES YOUR SKIN HEALTH AND MINIMIZES APOPTOSIS (CELL-DEATH)

Apoptosis is defined as the programmed death of a cell which occurs as part of the cell's normal activities.

But one may wonder how apoptosis is related to autophagy. Scientists believe that autophagy is a highly selective process by which a particular organelle(s) are eliminated from a cell. Also, there is tangible evidence to prove that one process does not control the other. However, there are reasons to believe that autophagy as a whole is a process of cell death that is independent of apoptosis.

Researchers are particularly interested in the association between autophagy and apoptosis because they believe that such knowledge could aid the treatment of cancer and management of neurodegenerative diseases such as Alzheimer's disease based on the capacity of both processes to regulate cell death. When such knowledge is available, autophagy could then be used as a therapeutic tool to eliminate harmful cells while protecting the healthy ones[7]

How to Induce Autophagy

Fossil evidence from the past showed strong and healthy bones and teeth of humans at an early age of our history, yet there are also evidences to show that most humans from ancient history went for days without food.

Some reasons responsible for this include:

- **They had to work to eat:** The early men had to farm or hunt before they could eat unlike today when you can easily stroll to a grocery store to buy foodstuffs.

- **They felt weak regularly:** Lack of energy is one of the primary triggers of autophagy

Here is a simple comparison between the ancient food environment and the modern food environment:

- **Most people have access to food:** Today, there is more than enough food for everyone to eat. Food is affordable and easily accessible to all.

- **People no longer have to work hard to eat:** Most of us drive down to the grocery or talk a short stroll down to the store with money in our pocket and VOOM, we can purchase high caloric food with a little amount of money. As a matter of fact, high caloric food items are the cheapest items on the shelf. We no longer have to farm or hunt before eating.

- **We can eat anytime we want:** If one is not cautious, you might find yourself munching one thing or another for most of the day.

In our modern-day society, an average individual can't go a day without taking in food substances that are capable of inducing autophagy. However, we do not engage in sufficient rigorous activities that could help expend energy to be energy deficient. In simple terms, our input is not equivalent to our output (i.e., what we take in does not equate what goes out). This is in sharp contrast with the eating environment in which our ancestors lived, and if they were given similar opportunity today, they would fall over each other to have a fill. In our modern society, the most important thing we need to focus on is finding ways to activate the process of autophagy.

Autophagy occurs in virtually all the cells in our body. However, this activity is further enhanced in response to stressful activities such as hunger, and starvation. Additional activities that could be considered as adequate stressors include exercise, fasting. Research has shown that both activities have helped to prevent age-related diseases, induce weight loss, and can extend the life-span of an individual.

Four ways of inducing autophagy while carrying out your normal daily activities:

1. Fasting. Due to our hectic lifestyles, it is good to know that you can still control your eating habits and your lifestyle. One of the good triggers of autophagy isn't very hard to imagine at all. One of the more popular triggers you can practice is intermittent fasting (IMF), and you can still take other liquids such as water and tea/coffee.

What is intermittent fasting? This is a form of time-restricted fasting in which an individual abstains from food for a specified period. We have different types of intermittent fasting such as the eating window and alternate-day fasting.

How long before autophagy is triggered? Well, studies have shown that fasting for 1-2 days (24-48 hours) usually produces the best effect.[8] However, this is an impossible task for most people. Still, many people can still fast for half a day (12 hours) or more without too much trouble, and this can be done by eating once or twice daily. For instance, if you had your last meal by 7 PM today, the next meal should come by 7 AM or thereabout. That way, you would have fasted for 12 hours. You could then have the next meal by 7 PM.

Another option is to have your regular meal at regular intervals then you go on a two to three day (2-3 days) fast. When it comes to alternate fasting, you could decide to cut down on your calorie intake during the fasting periods by eating only 1-2 meals (≤500 calories) then you can have your fill of calories on regular days.

Autophagy Fasting

Our bodies see any form of fasting as stress, and this sounds logical when you give it a bit of thought. During a fasting period, you feel hungry, and your body will attempt to maximize the distribution of your energy.

Below are the different kinds of fasts you can pick.

- **Long Fasts.** These type of fasts require you to stay away from any form of eating for a minimum of 24 hours.

- **Dry Fast.** This is a brutal form of fasting which remains popular despite its harshness. It is a hazardous form of fasting where you can't eat or drink anything. It is not advisable to stay away from drinking water; therefore, I would advise you to stay away from this type of fast for your health's sake.

- **Water Fast.** Water Fasting is another popular fasting type (and the reason for this book). This form of fasting is known for its autophagous, weight loss, detox, and anti-aging benefits. It requires you to stay away from eating but recommends you drink water or other forms of liquid depending on the variation of water fasting you are attempting. However, drinks such as protein shakes or juice are a "No" for it because they contain calories that could lead you to retain your weight.

Long fasts can enhance autophagy and weight loss. The loss of function by a stem cell can be reversed by one 24-hour fast, significantly improving their regeneration abilities.

You are probably thinking how long it will take you to fast to induce autophagy. Different research has shown that a fasting period of 24 to 36 hours would induce autophagy, suggesting that intermittent water fasting is another good option, although not as reliable as long water fasts, although

Fasting is about staying away from calories, to enable your body to reset its metabolic activities. This, however, doesn't mean you stay away from drinking water or specific teas, provided you don't add sugars, or you're selective about the natural sweeteners you add.

2. Ketogenic diets. Ketogenic diets (KD) are food substances that are very rich in fat but low in carbohydrates. Taking KD produces similar effects as fasting. KD comprises more than 75% of your daily fat consumption and less than 5-10% of calories obtained your daily carb consumption. When this is consumed, it triggers the body to undergo the process of gluconeogenesis (a process in which the body derives energy from non-carbohydrate sources such as fat).

Some food suggestions for KD includes eggs, avocado, fermented cheeses, seeds, nuts, butter, olive oil, fish, vegetables, vitamins, etc.

Ketone bodies are produced in response to KD which has several protective advantages. Multiple research works have shown that autophagy induced by starvation has neuro-protective advantages. For instance, the result of a study showed that rats fed with KD diets experienced a lesser amount of brain injury during a seizure.

3. Exercise. Exercise is one of the best stressors that are capable of triggering autophagy. One good thing about exercise according to reports from scientists is that it can trigger autophagy in many organs at the same time such as the liver, the muscles, the pancreas, the adipocytes, etc

Exercise helps the body regenerate and produce new tissues by breaking down worn out tissues and stimulating the body to create new ones. However, the amount of activity needed to stimulate autophagy is not yet clearly defined. For instance, 30 mins of exercise is enough to trigger autophagy in cardiac and skeletal muscles.

4. Sleep

Even though a vast majority of people replace rest time with binge-watching television, doing more work, and hanging out with friends, our body works at it's optimum when we acknowledge it's circadian rhythm or natural biological clock. This clock is in control of our sleeping cycles, as well as controls the process of autophagy.

It is vital to respect our circadian rhythm because it controls metabolic activities in the body. During our sleep, hormones are produced and released in our bodies. The absence of rest and sleep is seen as a stressful and distressing activity, and it negatively affects our health.

Sleep is therefore crucial in inducing autophagy as an absence of it alters the process of autophagy, and significantly slows it down.

Water-Fasting, Autophagy, and Anti-Aging The Intersection

Aging is a result of a decrease in the rate and amount of autophagy, leading to accumulation of higher amounts of junks and cellular damage.

As organisms age, they experience a decrease in their autophagous capacities which means that they cannot service and repair themselves as they used to any longer. As a result of this, there'll be an accumulation of cell damage, and after some time (days or months or years), most of the cells become damaged or malfunctioning, losing their ability to function at an optimal level. If this degradation gets to vital organs, death becomes inevitably close.

Autophagy occurs in a cycle, fluctuating at different rates at different times of the day. An increased level of eating reduces autophagy, while fasting increases it.

Therefore, if the result of aging is a decreased rate of autophagy and an increase in damage accumulation, and the effect of fasting is an increased rate of autophagy, then fasting combats aging.

Anti-aging is the greatest significant benefit that comes with water fasting. Water fasting is, in fact, the most effective anti-aging strategy available. Therefore, anything that enhances autophagy can have anti-aging effects.

We won't enter a fasting state if we eat food every time, and will in principle, never speed up autophagy.

Remember, eating constantly, or "grazing" is a pro-aging activity, so, don't eat all the time.

CHAPTER 7: WHAT ACTIVATES AUTOPHAGY?

This book isn't just about autophagy and what it is from a scientific or biological perspective. The purpose of this book is to show you how you can gain awareness of your own body intelligence to activate the power of your healing ability. It is amazing that we all carry this wisdom deep within our cells, yet most people have no knowledge of this process or why it is important to create opportunities for increased autophagy.

Once you understand the methods for activating autophagy, it is easy to consider bringing it into the fold of your regular diet, exercise, and lifestyle. If you have the knowledge to heal yourself, what would stop you?

So many people are surprised at the idea that we have the mechanisms to prevent and heal our illnesses and diseases. How we have spent the past hundred years, or so, is a direct link to the areas of our history that need attention. Not all science is fact. Some research has come and gone, having been disproven by new discoveries. We see it as a line in the sand when a group of researchers determine something new about long-held wisdom in the medical community. Crossing into the health lines of all, the research shows that one thing hasn't changed in our history as human beings, and that is our cellular design.

The basis of our survival across centuries hasn't come from the fad diet or the present-day version of correct exercise; we all have the understanding deep within us to prevent disease, and yet we can't help but struggle with the reality that men and women across the world are suffering from diseases. If you consider the ancient civilizations of men and women who foraged and hunted, you see that there wasn't any evidence of these illnesses. People might have had incurable ailments or severe injuries that caused an early death; however, cancer was not something detected in any archeological findings of human remains.

Piecing together the common denominators, what do we find? Serious illness isn't all inside us; it comes from everywhere outside of us—our choice of hamburgers and frozen pizza over kale and apples, our addiction to over-the-counter medications that only help you endure the symptoms but not cure the cause, our desire to relax on the couch with a TV show and stay inside with our cell phones, rather than go out for an evening stroll and enjoy the weather. All of these factors are outside of our bodies, and we are the one deciding to create these serious illnesses.

Facing the reality that you are causing your own illness isn't easy for anyone, and letting go of the sugar addictions, coffee habits, and favorite snack foods between meals has its challenges when your body is used to being fed these chemicals regularly.

What you can do to heal yourself is easy; all it takes is an eagerness to try. Because we have the internal body intelligence to heal, we need to know how to allow for that healing to begin. Thanks to the benefits of creating autophagy in our cells, we can now see what it is that is really kicking us into a position of cleansing and renewal.

There are several ways to activate this self-eating/self-healing process. A few of them all together prove to be most beneficial, allowing for a balanced, autophagic occurrence. When you start to ignite the process, you will understand the connection between each method of activation and how the healthier approach to stabilizing an autophagic detox will utilize several ways together. Like the cogs and wheels all working together to tell time.

Understanding each method separately will allow for a more fine-tuned, intentional approach to autophagy. It is important when activating this method of deep cellular healing that you attend to it carefully and healthily. Electing to use each method during your intentional autophagic activation, will provide you with the best results for internal repair and deep healing.

This chapter will approach each method and explain the how and why of each method as a source of autophagic initiation. Further chapters in this book will give more step by step guidance on performing these methods for increased autophagy.

Ways to Initiate Autophagy

Their are multiple ways by which autophagy is activated in both plants and animals that occur in the natural world without design or purposeful initiation. When your body is operating optimally, autophagy is occurring optimally also. In our current culture, the air we breathe, the water we drink, the multiple meals a day full of carbs, sugars, stimulants, and highly processed materials default our bodies to a setting of low performance. The elegant autophagic dance within cannot occur properly under such conditions, and in order to return to balanced levels of regularly occurring autophagy in our cells, we must begin by initiating the process and using the methods of activation to assist our bodies in healthy cell regeneration.

Before you get started with preparing to activate autophagy intentionally, it is important to understand how and why the methods outlined in this chapter work to promote that process. The major methods that will be discussed and detailed in this chapter are exercise, ketosis fasting, and intermittent water fasting.

Exercise
The benefits of exercise are long proven to establish a healthy, balanced body. The effects of exercise on all systems of the body are profound, and autophagy is part of the reason for this. The stress you put on your muscles when you exercise brings about the activation of autophagy. There are a variety of ways to exercise,

and some of them create a deeper impact on the cellular level than others. Exercise is also a large part of a smooth detoxification process. When you exercise, you increase your heart rate which pushes more fresh, oxygenated blood at a faster rate through your body, allowing for a swifter push and release of toxins coming out through a fasting or detox process, kind of like flushing the toilet.

With certain kinds of exercise, you can create a more impactful autophagic response, and coupled with some of the other methods, you bring about greater change and more abundant cell regeneration, upwards of 300% from if you weren't exercising at all, according to some research.

Ketosis

The process by which the body relies on fat stores for energy rather than sugars and carbohydrates is known as ketosis. More specifically, when certain foods are eliminated from the diet, the body turns to stored fats to burn as fuel. When the fat is used as energy, acids are left behind in the blood and are eliminated in the urine. These acids are known as ketones and are the indicator that you need to assure that fat is being burned.

Restricting calories in the diet and eliminating certain foods such as carbohydrates and sugars that turn into glucose, can stimulate the autophagic process by bringing about the change in cells through diet and ketosis.

Fasting

Fasting hasn't lost its mainstream impact since the dawn of early humans who scavenged the Earth for food. As we evolve, we can connect the dots more and more about certain methods of health and healing and the correlation with our early ancestors. Refraining from and restricting certain foods and eliminating them altogether, create an internal survival gateway to boost your body's need to stay alive until your next meal.

This connection to autophagy is what truly eliminates the wastes and toxins. As your diet becomes less involved, fewer meals and longer time between them, you instigate the action of cell renewal throughout the body systems. When you disengage from food for fuel, your body can rely on fat for fuel and give your cells an opportunity to clean house, so to speak.

Positive performance autophagy requires initiation through some food elimination and fasting. There are healthy methods and approaches as well as risks and dangers, so it will be important to have a handle on proper fasting methods before jumping in.

Intermittent Water Fasting

Along the history of humankind's search for food in times of foraging and hunting, at times, the only thing available was water. In today's health news, everyone insists on 8 glasses of water as the essential minimum requirement. The internal essence of every part of you, every muscle, organ, fiber, and cell, is water.

What you gain from fasting from food is an activation of autophagy; the goal of which is to recycle cell waste and rejuvenate the body from the cellular level. What you lose in the fasting process is water. Upwards of 30% of your daily water intake comes from food. When you take food away, you replace it with water. That is the basis of water fasting.

Intermittency is the timing of fasting for healthy, balanced autophagic performance. It will obviously cause irreparable damage to the body if you fast too long, too frequently. Fasting for short term periods is a healthy way to reestablish cellular function, and should be done alternating between eating a healthy diet and igniting autophagy with fasting.

As you can see, each method has its value and purpose in initiating autophagy. Together, these methods bring about cell renewal and regeneration, elimination of toxins, and prevention of disease. In the next sub-chapters, we will dig deeper into each method, assuring that you can healthily support autophagy for healing the cells.

Exercise

What happens to your body when you exercise? The answer lies on a deep, cellular level, not just in the physical results. Since early human existence, we have had to adapt and perform using our bodies to leverage the entire experience. Our bones, muscles, and tissues are what support us, keep us upright, and help us handle all activities in our everyday lives. Regardless of whether you are a caveman or a bank teller, you are using your muscles, bones, joints, and tissues, all of which are made up of tiny cells, specifically designed to function for each body process.

Early man had a greater need and opportunity to have regular exercise; it was the only way to survive. Before the advent of automobiles, factories, industry, and technology, human beings were required to use their bodies all the time, every day to accomplish the ins and outs of human existence. An exercise wasn't something you had to plan or schedule. Gym memberships were not a necessary part of reality. Life was exercise unless you were royalty and could lay around all day and eat decadent food to your heart's content, or rather discontent.

To understand the need for exercise on your body, you must look deep within the muscles and understand them on a cellular level. Bringing into focus the structure and function of your muscles, will bring you closer to understanding how autophagy can have an impact on this system, and why you want to create autophagy to heal this part of yourself.

Muscle is considered a soft tissue. It is found in most animals. Muscle cells are made of protein filaments that contain actin and myosin. These protein filaments glide past one another, creating contractions that change the length and the shape of the cell. Think of a bulging bicep: the muscle fibers collectively bulge to produce that shape when a certain action occurs. Force and motion are the functions of muscles. They have many roles such as moving your body in various ways, posture, internal organ movements like a heartbeat, and peristalsis, which is the movement of the digestive organs to move food through the body.

Myogenesis is the process by which the mesodermal layer of embryonic cells creates muscle tissue. The muscles can be divided into three types: striated (skeletal), smooth, and cardiac. The action of the muscle is either voluntary or involuntary. Involuntary muscles do not require conscious thought to function; they just perform their tasks, and you don't even realize it. The beat of the heart in cardiac muscle and the peristalsis of the intestines are examples of involuntary muscle movement. Skeletal or striated muscled requires conscious thought to move and is therefore called voluntary muscle movement. There are fast and slow twitch fibers when talking about skeletal muscle.

Oxidation of fats and carbohydrates is what powers muscles to make them move. Fast twitch fibers in skeletal muscles also use anaerobic chemical reactions. The reactions of the chemicals are what produced ATP, and adenosine triphosphate is what gives energy to the movement of the myosin heads in the muscle fibers.

The epimysium is a layer of tough connective tissue that sheaths the skeletal muscles. This tough tissue is what pins down the muscle tissues to the tendons. Bundles of fascicles lie within the epimysium, each one containing anywhere from 10 to 100 or more muscle fibers, all sheathed by another layer of tissue called perimysium. The perimysium is a pathway for nerves and blood flow to your muscles. Myocytes are the muscle cells and are like bundles of threads, encapsulated in its own collagenous endomysium tissue. The overall muscle is made up of all these tiny fibers that are all bundled together in fascicles to form your muscles. Every muscle is built of muscle cells.

Muscle function is supported by the membranes that surround each bundle, giving the energy and stamina it needs to resist passive stretching and maintain active performance.

Each muscle cell contains myofibrils. These are also bundled protein filaments and are complex strands of a variety of filaments that form to create sarcomeres. Sarcomeres are like candy canes, striated due to the intermittent layout of the skeletal and cardiac muscle. Actin and myosin are the filament components of the sarcomere.

There are significant differences between the three types of muscle, yet they all have the same cell function provided by the actin and myosin. The actin and myosin are what create the contraction of the muscle on the cellular level. The contraction of skeletal muscle on the cellular level is controlled by nerves that send electrical impulses from the brain, specifically, motoneurons (also cells). There are internal, pacemaker cells that are responsible for the involuntary movement of the cardiac and smooth muscles. The chemical neurotransmitter acetylcholine is what facilitates all skeletal and most smooth muscle contraction.

Movement of almost every muscle is decided by the origin and insertion of that muscle: where it comes from and what it attaches to. However, many sarcomeres are able to operate in a cross section of muscle determines the amount of force it can generate; the bigger your muscles, the thicker the sarcomeres, the greater the force. Every skeletal muscle is made of myofibrils, each one a chain of sarcomeres. The muscle cell contracts as one unit of sarcomeres, shortening simultaneously and lengthening simultaneously.

Leverage mechanics determines the amount of force that can occur in the action of the muscles in the external environment. An example of this would be flexing your biceps muscle.

Much of the body's energy consumption is through the movement of your muscles. Every muscle cell produces ATP which is the energy compound that creates the power to move the myosin heads in every muscle fiber. There is a short-term store of energy know as creatine phosphate, and it is born from the ATP. It can also regenerate ATP when it is needed with the compound known as creatine kinase. Muscles will also keep a store of glycogen, which is a form of glucose. It can be quickly turned into glucose when there is a need for sustained energy during incredibly powerful muscle contractions.

The molecule of glucose can be broken down anaerobically during glycolysis. Out of glycolysis 2 ATP and 2 lactic acid molecules are formed; however, this outcome is not produced in the aerobic state. Each muscle cell also has fat molecules that are utilized as energy during aerobic exercise. It takes longer to produce ATP in aerobic energy systems and requires more involved steps, yet it produces a great deal more ATP than what is seen in anaerobic glycolysis.

On another note, cardiac muscle can regularly consume all of the macronutrients listed above: protein, glucose, and fat. It can do this aerobically, as it is always working and pumping blood throughout the body. Also, the cardiac muscle will always take out the maximum amount of ATP from any involved molecule. These muscle fibers, as well as the liver and red blood cells, often consume lactic acid that is usually put out by the skeletal muscles during exercise; in essence, exercise helps the cells of your heart function.

Human muscle efficiency has been measured at up to 18-26%. This ratio comes from a breakdown of the output of mechanical work against the total metabolism, calculated from the consumption of oxygen. Low efficiency comes from a lowered generation of ATP from your food energy intake, and also the loss of converting ATP into mechanical action within the muscle fibers, as well as overall mechanical loss within the body. The loss of efficiency depends on the type of exercise being performed and the type of muscle fibers being used.

Having an understanding of the cellular function of muscles is vital when you are considering the way autophagy works. To break it down, muscle is the result of three, important things:

1. Physiological strength = size of the muscle, cross section of muscle, response to training
2. Neurological strength = the strength of signal given to the muscles telling them to contract (strong or weak signal)
3. Mechanical strength = force, leverage, joint capability

Discovering the lessons within the cells brings you face to face with the commitment, to knowing the inner workings of the cell's ability to not only perform their functions but also their ability to heal. The fine tuning that occurs deep within comes from the sophisticated machinery that makes up your entire being the cell. Muscle cells are as in need of autophagy as any other part of your body. Your muscles are your body, and if your muscle cells are unable to renew, then you lose the quality of function that keeps you feeling young and agile.

The vitality of out muscle health begins in the cell, like with all other systems in the body. One of the significant ways to activate autophagy is through the exercise of the muscles. Seeing the muscle up close helps you understand what is happening deep within when you exercise. The cells need cleansing so that your body can perform optimally. If you never exercise, how can your muscle cells do the work they are intended to do?

As we have engineered ways to unload the burden of labor onto machines and technology, we have accrued a need to find our daily dose of exercise in other ways. Many people have given up on exercise altogether, living in a culture that promotes a sedentary lifestyle in front of a TV, or a need to work for 8 hours straight sitting at a computer.

Our bodies need exercise to function well, and this has been proven over and over again. Benefits of exercise are far-reaching and here are a few examples:

- Good for muscles and bones—building and maintenance and the release of hormones to absorb amino acids in muscle and bone.
- Increased energy levels
- Reduced risk of chronic disease—improved insulin use, reduction of belly fat which leads to Type II diabetes, improved cardiovascular health, hormonal

balance, oxygen-rich blood to improve the vital function of all body systems.

- Weight loss—there are three ways to lose weight: digestion, body functions like breathing and heartbeat, and exercise. Exercise increases your metabolism and when combined with the right diet promotes weight loss.
- Improved brain health, memory and cognitive function—hormonal stimulation as well as oxygen-rich blood help the brain function optimally.
- Improved skin health—Your integumentary system is your largest organ and is an organ of elimination. Releasing toxins through the skin from exercise and sweating, can have a profound impact on the overall health of the skin.
- Pain reduction—Exercise provides a regulation of all body systems, enhancing the performance of cellular function allowing for the release and regulation of inflammation in the body which causes pain.
- Sleep regulation—regular exercise has been proven to aid your ability to sleep well. Physical exertion gives your body the opportunity to burn the energy in your body from all of the food you ate throughout the day. If you do not exercise and continue to consume calories, your body will want to burn the caloric

energy in some way, keeping you awake or restless through the night so that the energy can be burned.
- Improved mood—Exercise releases serotonin in the brain which is the happy hormone. Your mood will feel more uplifted and happier as a result of exercise.

The one completely overlooked aspect of all the benefits of exercise is that autophagy links to each benefit, causing the outcome to occur. What we feel or see on the outside as increased energy, happier mood, healthier body, and better sleep is the direct result of autophagy.

Every single cell in your body is contacted during the exercise experience. When you look at all of the cells operating as a whole universe of information and regulation, you can see how exercise can benefit not only the muscles and bones but every activity and function of the human body brought out by the action of autophagy. Exercise increases positive stress levels in the body. The act of engaging the muscles, skeleton, joints, ligaments, and tissues through specific motions causes fatigue in the fibers and even microscopic tearing. Even further in depth, the tears ask for repair through the sophistication of the cellular system, activating and increasing autophagy.

You certainly can create an autophagic response in the cells without exercise; however, for a balanced and healthy experience of healing the body, exercise will always be of benefit to you.

Variations on the kinds of exercise and levels of intensity are encouraged and recommended. Overuse of any muscle group or excessive weight lifting can also cause internal damage. It is a fine line to walk, so make sure you know what you are doing before you hurt yourself with exercise. Finding a balance with exercise styles will help improve and regulate autophagy, especially in combination with the other methods for activating this process.

Ketosis

Caloric intake in our early days as humans was highly limited. Agriculture wasn't invented yet and people hunted and gathered to survive, covering large distances regularly and fasting between meals. Typical diets were plants, seeds, nuts, fruits, and occasionally meats that were successfully hunted. Animal protein and fat were like drinking at an oasis after a long journey through the desert; it was what the body was ready for after a low calorie to no calorie intake and would replenish the body for more long distances ahead.

So, what does all of this mean? To break it down simply, ketosis occurs on the cellular level when you are low on glycogen in the body due to a lack of calories or a low carbohydrate diet. Your body burns fat through a sophisticated response and call of the chemicals in your cells. Everything is about balance on the microscopic level.

Ketosis is in balance when the body can burn stored fats. If the body has no fat reserves, or there is no fat being ingested, the body will feed on the proteins or muscles. When your body's insulin is not effectively utilized due to damaged, fatigued and dirty cell waste, ketones can accrue in the body creating a highly acidic internal landscape that can lead to illness and sometimes chronic disease. High acid inside the body is detrimental long term and requires a more balanced pH through the foods you eat, how much water you drink, and your vitamin and mineral intake.

High acid from ketones is known as ketoacidosis and is most often seen in people with diabetes who have issues with insulin regulation. It can also occur in extreme athletes who are overexerting their bodies over long periods with no caloric intake. Think of a triathlete trying to make it to the end of the race after the intensity of the exercises with little to no food. They can also experience ketoacidosis. Another example is childbirth. If a mother is laboring for days without eating, her body can start to react in this way.

Insulin and Ketosis

It is important to understand the role of insulin in ketosis. Insulin is produced in the pancreas, and it is energy, pure energy. Your body's cells use it to regulate proper intake of sugars in the body to operate efficiently. If your cells cannot receive proper doses of insulin, it will be rejected by the cell and end up in the bloodstream. Hyperglycemia is often a result of insulin production that can't release into the cells which chronically occurs and turns into diabetes.

What happens when your insulin production and intake are not effective or functional, is that your energy stores cannot regulate either. And the release of insulin in the blood creates acid or ketones, that lead to an overactive state of ketosis in which you are no longer burning fat. The body holds the fat, keeping you overweight, and starts to lock onto proteins, like the muscle. The exit of ketones from your body occurs through urination, and when you get tested for levels of ketones, it is your body's alert system that you are experiencing functional or dysfunctional insulin uptake due to a chronic overabundance of sugar in the blood. Your body doesn't know how to handle this, so systems begin to malfunction on a deep cellular level.

Here are some important facts you should know regarding insulin:
- Insulin resistance increases your risk of getting diabetes.
- You might be insulin resistant for years and not even know it.
- Insulin resistance usually doesn't trigger any obvious symptoms.
- The American Diabetes Association (ADA) has suggested that *up to fifty percent* of people with insulin

resistance and prediabetes will develop type 2 diabetes if they don't change their diet, exercise, and other lifestyle factors.
- Insulin resistance can *increase the risk* of obesity or being overweight, *high triglycerides*, high blood pressure.
- Insulin resistance may develop a skin condition in some people known as *acanthosis nigricans*. It looks like *soft, dark patches* sometimes on the back of the neck and armpits.
- A buildup of insulin within skin cells can cause acanthosis nigricans.

You may not be anywhere close to having diabetes; however, insulin resistance over time can lead to prediabetes and eventually type 2 diabetes. Seeing a doctor is the best option, and autophagy can be an added aid in preventing insulin resistance, that leads to diabetes and turning current diabetes around for the better.

Diabetes symptoms:

- Extreme thirst or hunger
- Having hunger, even after having just eaten
- Increased and/or frequent urination
- Tingling sensations in hands or feet
- Excessive fatigue
- Having infections often

There are tests you can take to test your blood sugar levels to find out if you are insulin resistant. The A1C test is the test given by a doctor to help measure your average blood sugar. It may be useful to get tested, so you have an idea of how autophagy can help you become less insulin resistant.

The test measurements look something like this:

- An A1C under 5.7 percent = normal.
- An A1C between 5.7 and 6.4 percent = prediabetes diagnoses.
- An A1C equal to or above 6.5 percent = diabetes diagnoses.

You can also have a fasting *blood glucose test*, which shows your fasting blood sugar level. This test is done after not eating or drinking for at least eight hours.

- Fasting blood sugar levels under 100 milligrams/deciliter (mg/dL) = normal.
- Levels between 100 and 125 mg/dL = prediabetes diagnoses.
- Levels equal to or greater than 126 mg/dL = diabetes.

A *glucose tolerance test* is another way to diagnose prediabetes or diabetes. Your blood glucose level is determined before this test begins, after which you receive a premeasured sugary drink. Your blood glucose level is then checked again 2 hours later.

- Blood sugar level after two hours of less than 140 mg/dL = normal.
- Result between 140 mg/dL and 199 mg = prediabetes.
- Blood sugar level of 200 mg/dL or higher = diabetes.

According to the American Diabetes Association, if you have insulin resistance, you may prevent diabetes by *exercising* 30 minutes, 5 days a week and eating a *balanced diet. Losing weight* can lower your risk of developing diabetes. Imagine what miracles you could work by activating autophagy.

Autophagy is the cleaning crew reaction that begins the change to reorganize cells for better insulin absorption. Without our insulin, the body's sugar levels would derail, and we would only eat off of our tissues. Thankfully, we all have insulin production coming from the pancreas, and can benefit the body by understanding how insulin works and how to regulate our diet and exercise, to allow for proper insulin sensitivity. For autophagy to correct this insulin dysfunction allowing for proper ketogenic performance, a resistance to foods can cause an internal turn of events that allows for proper cell function, namely cell clean-up.

Letting the cells control the dynamic inner world brings about the best body performance. Focusing energy inside the cell, autophagy consumes a great build-up of waste materials that causes the insulin resistance that leads to detrimental disease, and possible ketoacidosis.

What you want from ketosis is a healthy burning of fat fuel. When you are relying on fat stores, you can maintain healthy weight loss and weight consistency. Ketosis is promoted through autophagy, and in order to allow for healthy ketosis, a certain diet must be applied and practiced allowing for fat burning and toxin release.

Complex carbohydrates and sugars are eliminated to renew proper insulin use, performance autophagy, and ketosis. Testing ketosis is a way you can observe if you have activated autophagy in your cells. You can purchase Ketone Strips that change color when applied to urine samples and demonstrate ketone levels in the body, ranging from no ketosis to healthy ketosis to ketoacidosis.

Engaging in the benefits of ketosis will help your body properly produce and utilize insulin and use fat stores for fuel which assists in healthy weight loss without losing muscle.

Fasting

What you don't eat won't kill you, but extensive fasting will starve you to death. There is a fine line to walk regarding fasting to encourage autophagy, and damaging your lifeline connected to food. In reality, no wonder drug can cause an autophagic response in the body. The only way to truly enact the self-eating mechanism of the cell is to deplete the energy in the body by eliminating food.

Your energy is stored in each and every cell inside your system of life. The chemicals produced to create energy in the body release as needed to perform various functions. What if you needed to end the cycle of calories your body receives every day in order to allow for better cell performance?

Fasting gains on autophagy. What this means is that as you reduce the number of calories you ingest in a day you kick start autophagy. While your body is doing less to digest food and circulate nutrients in your body, creating new forms of energy, the cells have a hiatus from exposure to added energy and materials to process and can function to ball up all the garbage and throw it in the recycling bin. It's hard to work in the cell, and most of us aren't thinking microscopically when we eat our daily bread.

Today's diet is extreme. Most Americans eat 3-square meals a day with snacks in between, coffee, sugar, additives, and highly processed foods that are chemically engineered in laboratories, as well as endless quantities of prescription drugs and over the counter medications. On top of all those toxins, the average American is chronically dehydrated, choosing sugary beverages over clean water. There is no way to effectively flush the toxins under those conditions.

What happens when you keep adding calories, limit exercise and refrain from regular water consumption? Disease, obesity, mental and physical stress, mental and physical illness, depression, anxiety, trouble sleeping, inflammation, and more.

When you realize the detrimental impact of the American diet on the cellular level, you begin to understand the chronic disease plaguing the nation. The answer is simple: fasting for autophagic performance.

When people think of fasting, they think of rail-thin, bony people who are making a religious or political sacrifice, like Gandhi or the suffragette, Alice Paul. They think of individuals who succumb to extreme dieting methods to lose weight, no matter the cost and end up with psychological disorders like Anorexia Nervosa and Bulimia.

Fasting for health is not starvation. There are limits to consider when approaching this method for activating autophagy. What you find, rather than severe loss of food intake and extreme measures of weight loss, is a carefully regulated and balanced approach to caloric restriction and food elimination. You do not eliminate it permanently; it is a temporary act to elicit the autophagic response.

Many fasts are only 16-18 hours, several days a week, while others may last 24-72 hours with healthy boundaries of when it is too long. Here are a few fasting methods to consider:

- Time-restricted—This will include a daily ratio of time that you are not eating and the time that you are. A common ratio is 16:8 whereby you fast for 16 hours and allow food for 8 out of the full 24-hour day. You can adjust the ratio as long as the fasting time is at least 16 hours for a maximum autophagic benefit.

- Alternate Day Fasting—Here, you will alternate days you eat with days you don't. Essentially, Monday you eat food; Tuesday you don't. Wednesday you eat food; Thursday you don't, etc.
- Intermittent Fasting—This is a full 24+ hour day fast separated by days or weeks. That could look like one day fast once a week or twice a month, or perhaps a 2-3 day fast once a month.
- 5:2 Diet and Fast—This ratio suggests eating for 5 days and fasting for 2 every week.
- Low-Calorie Fast—This kind of fast includes an extreme reduction of calorie intake over a period of time but still allows for some calories to be ingested.
- Religious or Political Fasting—This is beyond the scope of this book; however, these kinds of fasts are important to the beliefs of some individuals. It is important that no matter the reason for the fast, you should see to it that you are doing it in a healthy, balanced way.

The basic tactic is to resist food long enough to promote autophagy. Permitting this small fasting time multiple days, a month, or year can reduce your body's cell deterioration significantly.

What you don't want to do, is extend the fast to the point that your body overextends ketosis which causes acidic cell damage, that can lead to fatality and bring about unnecessary starvation, that causes the body to eat muscle rather than fat stores. This is why engaging in short-lived fasting can provide autophagic cell renewal, while burning fat and restoring optimal cell function.

Dieting has been proven to benefit in the short term; however, most people try to trick their bodies into losing weight without engaging in autophagy and ketosis. While some diets can be useful under certain conditions and for certain ailments, a majority of mainstream diets lead to insulin resistance, weight retention, and problematic sugar highs and lows that lead to binge eating.

Waste in the cells can easily accumulate under these conditions and without autophagic response initiation, the waste will build, the cells will operate at a dysfunctional or slow level, and balanced health will not be fully restored. Fasting improves the body's ability to restore itself. Taking short breaks from food intake has been scientifically proven to activate autophagy, which allows the cells in your body to clean up and reorganize, leading to a fresher, healthier, more youthful you.

In addition to the overall health benefit of food fasting, research is also showing that autophagy induced by fasting, has an impact on the healing of chronic illness and disease. There have been reports that creating this response in the body while battling cancer, diabetes, and inflammatory diseases can allow for deeper, cellular healing and prevention of future recurrence of the illness that cannot be remedied by prescription drugs, chemotherapy, or surgery.

This is your body intelligence at its finest. We are sophisticated machines that have the capability to self-heal, and creating the autophagic process through careful, healthful fasting could very well save your life.

Intermittent Water Fasting

Water is life. No cell in your body can function without it. No living thing on Earth can exist without water's vital essence. Because performance autophagy relates to cell tissue cleansing and renewal, without water, this process would be null and void. The basic human cell is protein, fat, cholesterol, and water. While you begin to increase autophagy through fasting and ketosis, you begin the process of reducing wastes and toxins in the body on a cellular level.

Water will get used to performing all these functions, collecting and disposing of exhausted materials and compounds. The point of energy is to give life to our experience. The point of water is to give life to that energy. Because water is so significant to the system as a whole, water fasting is a described method of autophagy on account of its ability to enhance autophagic reaction and response.

Timing is everything. Intermittence is a level of time which allows your body to receive ample energy through healthy eating and diet, followed by moments and periods of fasting. This alternating effect brings about effective autophagy, giving space and time to the cells to renew and for the body to gain nutrients; both are necessary for optimal health.

Water fasting is the method by which all food is eliminated slowly over the course of several hours and/or days to allow your body time to gently respond and react to fewer calories. Water is then increased to allow for proper autophagic response and activity. The only thing consumed in water fast is water; however, some vitamins and minerals may be consumed for proper internal balance. Although no calories are ingested, some vitamins and minerals are necessary for the proper function of the cells so that they may do their work during autophagy.

Water is essential; it carries all life and acts as the conduit of all internal function and performance. Without it, autophagy wouldn't work. Balancing the fast with extra water is key to healthy autophagic response and brings about greater change, renewal and deep cellular healing.

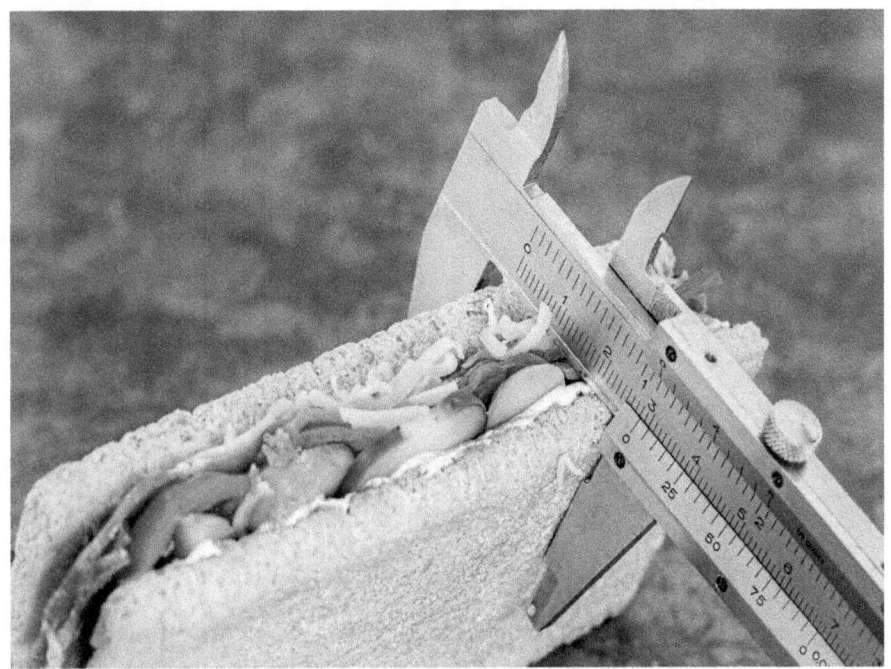

CHAPTER 8: HEAL YOUR BODY FROM WITHIN

Autophagy is a process which can be induced by different factors. This chapter will not cover the pathways of autophagy AMPK and mTOR, but it will cover instead how to induce it, how to plan it in real life. As previously mentioned in this book, autophagy can be favored by Intermittent Fasting, Ketosis, HIIT, Protein Fasting and Sleep.

How To Make Fasting A Way of Life?

Becoming healthier and more fit should be a primary goal that anyone should follow. Autophagy can help you achieve this goal, as it's responsible for destroying and recycling old and damaged cells parts, in order for your body to work better. It is usually linked with the fat burning process, as autophagy happens when the body runs on fat. It basically actions on the fat cells, in order to get the energy required for your brain and body. Ketosis and fasting can be intertwined, as ketosis is regarded as the first phase of Intermittent Fasting, during which ketones levels are higher. Ketosis is not the same thing as the keto-adaption process. The first term describes a metabolic state with appropriate levels of ketones and blood sugar. During this phase, the insulin level and blood sugar decreases, whilst the ketones levels are increasing. This is generated by the glucose deprivation, meaning that it took quite a while since the body last had its glucose required for energy. This substance can be found in all the carbs (and proteins as well) and is the primary source of energy for the body under "normal circumstances." Speaking of glucose intake, the modern-day diet relies heavily on carbs because we mainly consume processed food. This means that the body mainly uses the glucose from the carbs, but the big problem is that it simply can't burn all the glycogen it gets, mainly because of the high carb intake, but also because of the passive lifestyle. Nowadays, around 70% of the diseases known to humans are caused by the food we eat, and high amounts of carbs can be blamed for this situation. In urban communities, where most people live, is kind of difficult to find natural and organic food, as everywhere you are bombarded by processed food. The sad truth is that most of the food we eat today is processed, and this comes with very high levels of carbs. What's even worse, is that these types of food have little to nothing nutritional value and causes addiction. In order to cover your daily nutritional needs, you have to eat more, but this means a caloric boom. Processed food is more caloric dense than nutrient dense, and this is a major disadvantage. When people are facing increased risks of chronical diseases like type 2 diabetes, heart, stomach, liver and kidney diseases, it's clear that something has to be done to change the way we eat and also what we eat. Studies indicate that in order to become healthier and also thinner, you would need to decrease the glucose level when eating. This can happen by cutting down on carbs and, in some cases, also means protein limiting. When not burned, glucose gets stored into your blood, increasing the insulin and blood sugar level. Carbs consumption is like a vicious circle, as you easily get hungry after consuming food rich in carbs, and you are craving for more. But these meals come with strings attached, as you will get higher glucose levels and eventually higher blood sugar and insulin level. In order to make a radical change, you will need to make your body burn fat, not glucose. As you probably already have blood sugar, you will need to stop eating so many carbs, and therefore you will have less glucose to worry about. You can achieve this through fasting (restraining yourself from food) or through a special diet.

Traditional fasting means not consuming any food at all; some would not consume anything at all, just like religious fanatics during a special period, the Ramadan in the Islamic religion can be a perfect example. By not consuming anything at all, you are allowing your body to use the available glucose to be burnt, and once it has burned it all, the body will have to switch the energy source from glucose to fat. As the glucose level is decreasing, the same happens with the insulin level, setting it free to do its job and regulate the blood sugar. The body easily adapts to such changes, and since its glucose reserves are running out, it has to figure out a way to use a different fuel type. That's where ketones step in, which is the necessary tool to break down fat cells and release the energy from them. You need to easily make the difference between ketosis and the keto-adapted process, as ketosis represent the metabolic state during which the ketone bodies are multiplying. The keto-adapted process is responsible for switching the energy source from glucose to fat. You can be in a ketosis state, but still not running on fats and ketones for fuel.

Intermittent Fasting is more of a self-discipline process because it's about planning when to eat than what to eat. Limiting the feeding window to a limited amount of hours can give time for the body to process the food and use it for energy. However, when the body has already processed the food it has consumed and it's not receiving anything else, it will start to look for a different alternative as fuel. The fat tissue is the most "to hand" option and ketones can help extract the energy from it. If daily fasting has feeding and a fasting window, these terms are not the same with the fed and fasted state. The fed state represents the period of time required by your body to process the food it consumed, whilst the fasted state refers to the period after the fed state, during which the body doesn't have to process any food, and it's also not receiving any nutrients at all. The fasted state starts approximately 12 hours after the last meal, and, coincidence or not, that's when ketosis starts. In the fasted state, the ketones levels are increasing rapidly, whilst the blood sugar and insulin levels are decreasing. At this point, the body doesn't have available glucose to burn, and it's looking for alternative fuel. Also, this is the right moment to apply stress to your body, and by stress, you need to understand the physical exercise. This will force the fat burning process, will increase even more the ketones levels and the insulin will take care of the stored glucose from your blood. This is how the keto-adaptation gets started when your body starts to run on fats. Since ketosis is considered the first phase of Intermittent Fasting, these 2 processes go "hand-in-hand," but ketosis can be achieved in a different way also, through a keto diet. Sticking to the IF process, if you want to achieve autophagy, you may need to fast for a longer period of time, as daily fasting may not be enough for autophagy. Fasting between 24 and 48 hours should normally induce autophagy, but this is not an exact science, as the fasting period required to trigger the autophagy period may be different from a person to another. Some people have tried fasting for a longer period, consuming just water. However, this method should only be tried as a last case scenario, as it can be pretty drastic to try it for a longer period of time. Most of the Intermittent Fasting benefits can be achieved after up to 72 hours of fasting, so there shouldn't be any reasons to fast longer than that. Autophagy will be triggered during this kind of fast, so you will get rid of the damaged proteins, organelles and cell parts from your body and replace them with brand new ones. If you are worried about muscle loss, I have news for you. The growth hormone reaches incredible levels after 72 hours of fasting, so you will not only burn fat, but you will maintain your muscle mass. Getting more muscle mass depends on the protein intake and the intensity of training. 72 hours fast will not get you the performance you are looking for, so you will not gain more muscles. You are not getting any proteins also, as you are consuming just water.

During the fasting process, you will have to train your brain to forget about food and to deal better with the hunger situations, as you will be experiencing starvation. There are softer fasting programs, which can also induce autophagy so you will not have to rush into the hardest one. You can try several of them, depending on the difficulty level of the program. Some fasting methods would include the Leangains method (16 hours of fasting correlated with 8-hour feeding window), The Warrior Diet (4-6 hours of eating time, the rest is just pure fasting), Eat Stop Eat (or the 24 hours fast) and the Alternate Day Diet (12 hours feeding window/36 hours fasting period). The "purest" method of fasting is considered water fasting, but this is usually a long term fast and very radical, as you can't consume any calories at all. Officially, the feeding window of any fasting program doesn't have any special food requirements. Practically, in order for the program to be more effective, you will need to cut down on carbs, so you simply can't eat anything you want. Food types like bread, pasta, pastries, potatoes or rice should be eliminated from your diet, or consumed in moderate amounts. You can try the daily fasting, or you can try fasting every other day or just once per week. Depending on your objective, you can select one of the available fasting programs. This procedure is not for everyone, so if you have a medical condition, perhaps Intermittent Fasting is not for you.

Another way to enter the ketosis phase is the keto diet; a special LCHF method focused on making your body run on fats. This type of diet replaces carbs with fats, so it lowers them to a minimum level, or perhaps just eliminates them completely. Intermittent Fasting mostly relies on starvation to induce autophagy. The keto diet relies on carbs deprivation to induce it. When it comes to carbs, you need to know that they are present in too many types of food, especially if it's processed. Carbs are divided into sugars in starch. Sugar is probably the most harmful ingredient on the face of the Earth. It's consumed at a global scale, and it has too many people addicted to it. The effects of sugar consumption are obvious for most people. Different governmental measures were taken in order to better inform the consumer of the risk of sugar, products are properly labeled so you can see the sugar level on it, and some governments have even applied an extra tax on products containing sugar. All of these measures were designated to lower the consumption of such products. Any processed product has a smaller or higher value of sugar, but there is a few which can be considered sugar bombs. You need to avoid consumption of soft drinks, fruit juices, sweets, candies and so on.

The other major carb type is represented by starch, which can be found in bread, pasta, pastries, rice, and potatoes. Moderate consumption, or even completely eliminating these types of food from the menu is desirable, although these types of food are amongst the most common and popular worldwide.

The keto diet significantly lowers the carb intake because they are the main source of glucose. However, glucose can be found in proteins as well, so lowering the protein level is also something that you need to do. The keto diet should have a ratio of just 5% carbs, 15% - 25% proteins and the rest should consist of fats. This is the standard keto diet. There is also a version which involves a higher protein intake, but not higher than 35%, but also keeping the carbs level extremely low. The keto diet is capable of inducing autophagy, although through it the body gets fed. Autophagy is induced when the body runs on fat, and this is where the keto diet steps in. If Intermittent Fasting trains the body to consume the fat reserves, the keto diet trains the body to use the fat consumed through this diet, and once that's finished, to continue consuming fats from the fat reserves.

As mentioned above, the keto diet focuses more on food types with higher levels of fat. That's why you will need to include in your menu food types like avocado, olive oil, fish (especially salmon), meat (pork, beef or chicken), eggs, high-fat dairy products, fruits, leafy green veggies, legumes, nuts, berries and so on. Avocado should be present in any keto diet, as it has plenty of benefits for the fat burning process and for autophagy itself. When it comes to fish, make sure you consume the fatty kind of meat, salmon is perhaps the best example. Tuna is also a good alternative. When it comes to meat, you can go for the fattier ones, but still, you will need to consume them moderately, as there are also sources of proteins and glucose. The same rule applies for fish as well. Eggs are highly recommended during a keto diet so you can consume as many as you like, but still don't exaggerate with them. High-fat dairy products should not be missing from any keto diet. You can consume in this case butter, yogurt, cream or cheese, all high fat. Milk is not quite recommended, as it's also a source of carbs, regardless if it is semi-skimmed or whole milk. When it comes to fruits, you can include most of the fruits known to man, especially oranges, limes, lemons, apples, pineapples, mango, kiwi and all sorts of berries, as they are known for inducing autophagy. In terms of vegetables, the general rule is what grows over the ground. So, you can use plenty of lettuce, green salad, spinach, cauliflower, broccoli, Brussels sprouts, but also celery, carrots, onions, garlic, peppers, asparagus and many more. Nuts are very good for a ketogenic diet, so you can consume all kind of nuts in this diet, but also moderately.

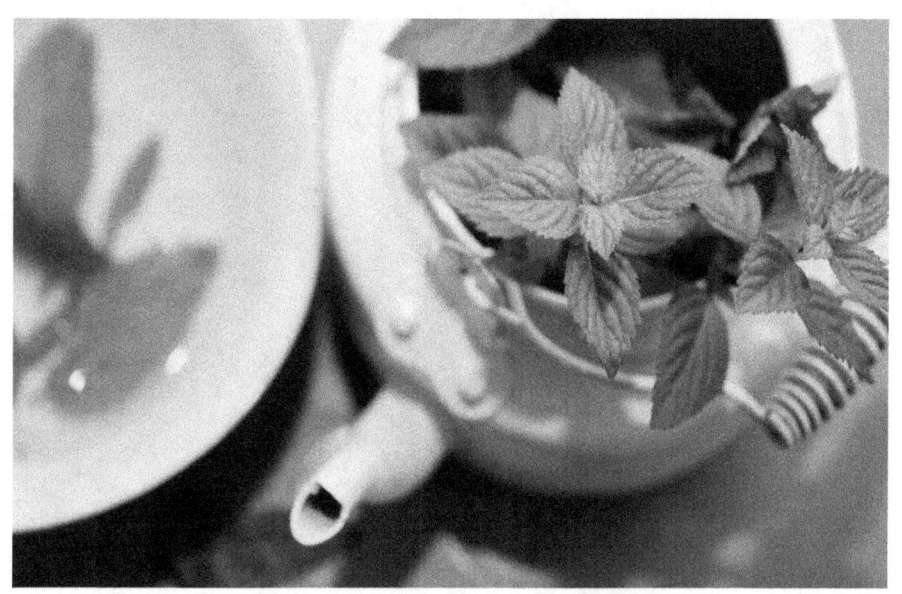

CHAPTER 9: WEIGHT LOSS

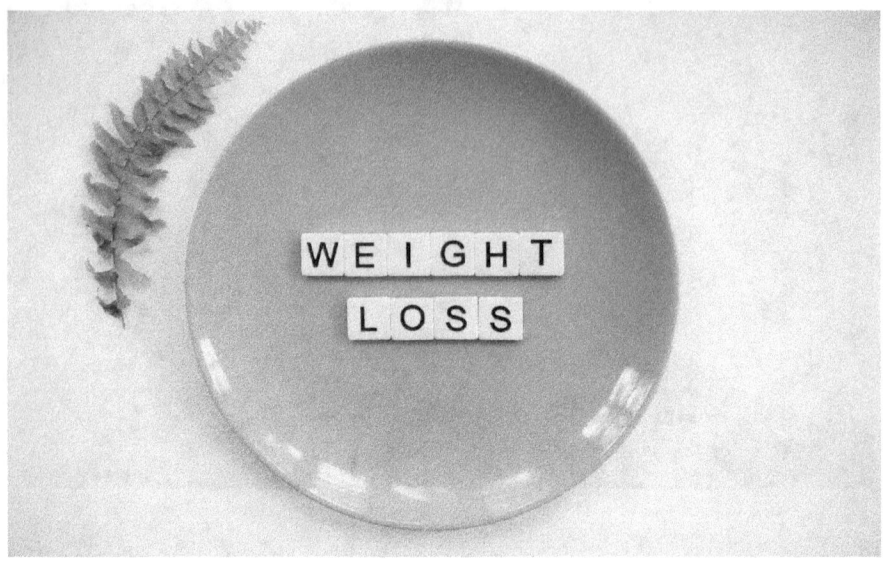

Hunger over the course of a water fast is greatly reduced when you start your fast off on the right foot. Energy may start off being lower during the fast, but the consumption of only water from 1-3 days restricts your caloric intake to allow for significant loss in weight. Because of the possible ketosis already occurring from the right diet, your body will already be burning fat stores over muscle allowing for healthy autophagic cell renewal.

What happens then is that during your short-term water fast, you are burning unwanted fat stores and flushing toxins from that stored fat with the water. The result is weight loss.

Loss of weight can get out of hand resulting in your body's instinct to control the loss of fat, hanging onto the reserves for survival.

This can lead to taking energy from the protein stores in the body, which is why it is important to balance the fasting with the right diet, right exercise and right rest.

Fasting is believed to be one of the most effective ways to induce autophagy because of the entrance into a state of stress. The stress of this kind relates to the body's ability to engage all systems for survival. When these systems are over-engaged and out of hand, it can lead to severe illness; however, when done properly, recurring periods of timed stress can activate the body's ability to collect and remove waste for the optimal function that allows for survival. This is body intelligence.

Weight loss occurs when you fast, and water fasting actually enhances the ability to flush out what is needing to be released, adding to the overall loss of weight. Effects of fasting, when done properly lead to steady, regulated weight loss.

With the slow transition back to food, you are able to maintain the new weight and experience the rejuvenation on the cellular level caused by autophagy through fasting. There is no current evidence to suggest that weight loss is unhealthy through fasting. When one is properly prepared for a fast, there is less potential for harmful side effects. What you lose in weight, you gain in health.

Weight loss is one of the main reasons people fast. You don't have to water fast only to achieve significant weight loss. You can apply any of the methods of fasting revealed in Ch. 2.4 to promote weight loss; however, the results of water fasting, consuming only water for a period of time, creates a more profound impact on the initiation of autophagy and promotes the flushing of toxins and ketones from the body.

If the goal with water fasting is weight loss in addition to autophagy, be sure to allow time to phase into the right diet. Try incorporating a ketosis diet for 2-4 weeks, or more, before you begin to incorporate fasting. You may already begin to notice significant weight loss from the keto-diet alone. After a period of weeks, or months, you may hit a weight loss plateau and can use water fasting as a kick start to achieve more weight loss. Once you have regulated your diet in this way, you can begin to create a deeper autophagic response by slowly reducing food and calorie intake to enter into a fasting period. Again, you can determine the right fasting method for you by listening to your body and paying careful attention to what works best for your body type, genetic history, and overall health.

Water fasting is an excellent method for promoting autophagic performance, which leads to healthy loss of weight that you can further maintain and regulate through right diet, exercise and rest.

CHAPTER 10: FEELING GOOD

Part of healing is allowing periods of time for your body to regenerate. Autophagy is a powerful, internal intelligence. Your body has the power to heal itself, but if you are not offering it the proper time to rest, you will be digging a deeper hole to clean up later.

Starting off on the right foot and creating good, healthy habits for wellness is essential to locking down the results you are looking for. In our current culture, everything is fast-paced, instantly gratified, and we are all plugged in all day long to our devices. Many people have 40-60 work weeks that make it challenging to find time for rest, let alone diet, exercise, and healthy fasting.

Bringing your health into focus includes allowing for proper periods of rest. During your experience in activating autophagy, it will be important to organize time for your body to rest. Rest is important after significant exercise. When you strain and stress your body, it requires time to recover and repair microscopic damage to the muscle fibers and tissues.

When you eat a meal that is filling, it is helpful to enjoy a period of rest after to allow your body the proper amount of time to digest. Your body can focus on digestion better if you offer it the rest to do so.

Fasting is something that can temporarily lower your energy since you are not ingesting any calories. It is common to experience some fatigue under these circumstances. It is a great opportunity to incorporate rest for your body while it is fasting. Imagine too, on the microscopic level, when you are resting your body is undergoing great healing, transformation and change, performing autophagic response from the intermittent fasting.

Many people consume large amounts of sugar and caffeine daily to bump them out of slumps that occur throughout the day, after meals, after long periods of work, or because of lack of sleep the night before. If you replace your caffeine and sugar doses with moments or periods of rest throughout the day, you would aid your body in a much healthier way, eliminating the need for caffeine and sugar altogether.

Sugar is the antithesis of a healthy diet and optimal autophagic performance and should be avoided anyway if you are planning on activating autophagy. Caffeine is regularly consumed by most people, and it is not discouraged in the majority of diets. The longer-term effects of daily caffeine intake can be as detrimental to your body as any other stimulant or toxin. Successful autophagic performance doesn't need caffeine and like other foods and beverages that hinder health. It should be avoided and replaced with herbal teas, water, and other non-caffeinated beverages.

You can ultimately rest better without it, and if you are getting the rest you need, you won't need caffeine at all.

The right rest comes with experimentation, awareness of your needs, listening to your body, and responding to it when it is asking for rest. Incorporating the right rest will fluctuate depending on day to day life, activities, exercise, diet, schedule, and more.

Rest is vital to supporting optimal autophagic performance. All four components together bring about a level of health, that will deliver clear results that you can see and feel. Activating autophagy through the combination of right diet, exercise, fasting, and rest are the key to a long and healthy life.

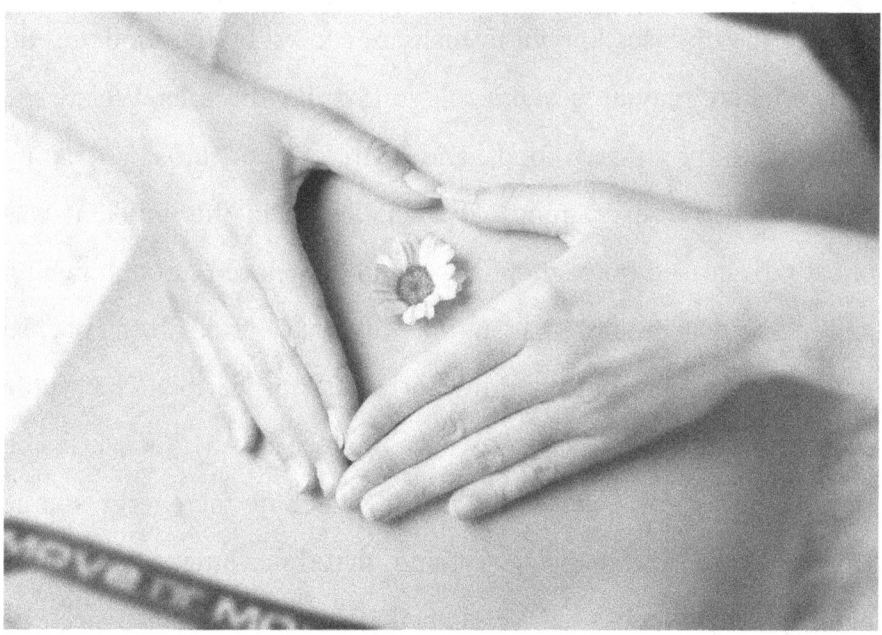

CONCLUSION

The researches on Autophagy deserved to win the Nobel prize in Physiology or Medicine in 2016, as it's a practice that revolutionizes the medicine. The process of recycling damaged parts of proteins and organelles at a cellular level can have plenty of benefits for the human body, in terms of health especially. Only when you think of several benefits that autophagy can have, like a better cognitive function (protecting you from neurodegenerative diseases like Alzheimer's and Parkinson's disease), lower blood sugar and insulin level (thus preventing type 2 diabetes), increased ketones level (favoring the fat burning process), appetite control and prevention of heart, kidney, stomach or liver diseases. Around 70% of the diseases known to man are caused by the food we eat, and carbs are playing a major role in favoring diseases. We are too exposed to processed food, and therefore to carbs, so eating healthy it's becoming more of a challenge. In this book, it was already discussed how autophagy could be induced through fasting and the ketosis process. Fasting literally means food abstinence, so you don't have to eat anything in the fasting period. The whole purpose of this process is to burn more fat. As glucose is the default fuel type for the human body, switching the energy source from glucose to fats is something that Intermittent Fasting is aiming for. Glucose is originated from carbs, but since we consume too many carbs and we have a sedentary lifestyle, it doesn't get burned by the body, so it gets stored in the blood, raising the insulin and blood sugar levels. By switching to fats, Intermittent Fasting forces ketones to multiply and to extract the energy from the fat cells. Whilst this happens, the insulin level is getting lower, and it takes care of the blood sugar, regulating it. Ketosis is a phase of Intermittent Fasting during which the ketones levels are significant increases, whilst the blood sugar and insulin level decreases. The Keto-Adaptation process is when the body starts to run on fats as the default fuel type. There are several ways of fasting and even a keto-diet, all of them favoring the autophagy process. However, if fasting is not your thing, you can induce autophagy through HIIT (a really intense workout) or through protein fast, which is a special one-day diet, which involves keeping the daily protein intake to less than 15 grams. Another important piece in the autophagy puzzle is sleep, as autophagy happens during sleep, so without proper restful sleep the whole process wouldn't take place. Combining all of these factors will get you a lot closer to autophagy.

www.ingramcontent.com/pod-product-compliance
Lightning Source LLC
Chambersburg PA
CBHW070649220526
45466CB00001B/359